FlatTop

Navigating Breast Cancer With Attitude, Fortitude & Spirit

Ideas & Musings

by Donna Wodianka

FlatTop

DEDICATION

For

Rachel, Joe, and Adam — my joy, my strength, my reason

&

Mary Jane, whose unflinching courage and irrepressible

spirit light the way for us all

FlatTop

CONTENTS

FlatTop

ACKNOWLEDGMENTS

If I tried to thank everyone who has made a difference in my cancer journey, I would fill this book and then some. Cancer is more than a personal, or even a family, disease; it calls on an entire community to come together and lend support. I thank every one of you, from the surgeons, specialists, nurses, and medical teams who so tenaciously square off with this disease every day to the family members, friends, colleagues, and neighbors who so generously share their love and compassion. My gratitude runs deep.

Special, loving thanks to:

My children, for filling my heart to bursting with love, light, and laughter —

Rachel, who has bravely navigated every leg of this journey right beside me

Joe, who keeps me laughing and inspired me to write this book

Adam, who helps me stay grounded and reminds me to always hear the music

… and in memory of Michelle, whose loving spirit touches our lives every day

My parents, Ardith and Paul, for teaching me everything I know about unwavering love, faith, and courage

My sister, Debbie, for never once letting go of my hand

My brother, Paul, for believing in me almost as much as I believe in him

My brother-from-another-mother, Tracy, for literally giving me the shirts off his back (old, worn-out flannel, but still)

My nephews, niece, great-nephews, and great-nieces, for always bringing me joy (and making me pictures!)

My dear cousins and friends, whose prayers, calls, gifts, and love have lifted and inspired me more times than I can count

Mary Jane, who showed me how it's done! (You are a *phenomenon*.)

Brad, who was truly my lifeline in the storm

Dr. Lois, for your selfless commitment to the cause (Why *don't* you wear a cape?)

My spiritual healing team - *Namaste*.

Preface
You Are Never Alone

We're not all cut out to be warriors. That doesn't mean we can't win "the fight."

One warm spring day as I walked around the block, bald head nestled in a scarf and complexion the color of the concrete beneath my feet, a neighbor called out, "Keep fighting!" I smiled and offered as much of a wave as I could muster. While I was deeply touched by his sentiment, I couldn't help but think that he was giving me much more credit than I deserved. It was true that I had weathered a bilateral mastectomy and was in the throes of chemo; radiation would be next. Also true: My doctors weren't entirely confident that these treatments would be enough to obliterate the cancer cells still lurking in my lymph nodes. So I was in it, for sure. But *fighting?* I wasn't fighting. I was just navigating the course that had been set out in front of me.

That's the thing about breast cancer: The media hype it up to be some kind of glorified contest between us and our disease. Were they to sketch it out, I imagine we would be engaged in hand-to-hand combat with this mortal enemy — cancer commandos armed with strength, guile, and agility belying our ever-present nausea and neuropathy. In this scenario, our prize, having ultimately "won the fight," is the lifelong right to cavort in the streets wearing pink T-shirts proclaiming us "survivors." A friend of mine, with the best of intentions, presented me with a survivor T-shirt, only this one had an additional message emblazoned on its front: "I'm my own hero." Really? I was embarrassed. I didn't want to hurt her feelings, so I just said thank you. What I wanted to say, though, was that I'm no hero, just a regular human person trying to save my own ass. That's sort of instinct, isn't it?

The problem that arises from all of the publicity is that we end up believing that we need to be superheroes to face this disease. That's a lot of pressure to put on ourselves, especially at a time when we feel so vulnerable.

So please trust me when I tell you that it's simply not true: You don't need superpowers to get through your cancer experience. Everything you need is already inside you. You may have to "dig deep," as the cliché goes, to bring it to the surface, but once you tap into it, it will be there any time you need it. What's "it"? A powerful combination of faith, an open mind, and a relentless sense of humor.

When I was diagnosed, I didn't get angry, didn't ask "Why me?," didn't shake my fist to the heavens even once. While I realize these would have been normal reactions to the situation — plenty of people fight cancer successfully with rage and indignation — this approach just didn't occur to me. I've never been the warrior type. I was of course shocked and saddened when I heard the diagnosis. But my instinct was to go *with* it rather than fight *against* it — in other words, to get my spirit in step with the healing process that is the natural protector of my body. My gut feeling was that if I could power up this very positive aspect of my being, I could move beyond this disease and regain my health.

For me, this approach worked not only in the long run but also as I approached each day during even the most intense stretches of time. Regardless of pain, nausea, fatigue, or other symptom of the moment, I would wake up each morning grateful for whatever level of health my body might have. I visualized myself vibrant and whole, and I set my intentions on that state of perfect health.

That's not to say that spiritual strength was the *only* factor in my healing equation; I'm of course infinitely grateful to the medical teams who unleashed their most powerful treatments on my cancer. But I know in my heart that if I had not gone into these treatments with a positive outlook and limitless faith, I would not be here today. So, while I would never promise to have all the answers or some miracle cure to share with you, I do hope that you can benefit from what I learned on my path so that you can walk confidently ahead on your own.

What's so funny? I mentioned the importance of having a sense of humor as you embark upon this journey, and while that might seem counterintuitive when contemplating the seriousness of this disease, humor has the power to bolster your spirit and renew your strength when you need it most. Honestly, people who have never had cancer themselves typically start squirming when you use "cancer" and "humor" in the same sentence. But people who *have* cancer generally appreciate comic relief. When I talk with my friends who have, or have had, cancer, we can laugh all day long about the ridiculous things we've experienced along the way.

For my family and me, laughter has always been good medicine. Cancer didn't stop that. In fact, it was my son Joe's sense of humor that gave me the idea to write this book. Here's what happened:

The weekend after I shared my diagnosis with my three amazing 20-something kids — Rachel, Joe, and Adam — we were driving to a restaurant together. I had a couple of weeks until surgery, and I wanted to spend some quality time together before the cancer adventure was in full swing.

Rachel, who was sitting in the back with Adam, had a cold. As she sniffled and coughed, looking sadly out the window, I decided to tackle the elephant in the room. "Rachel! Are you sulking back there about a silly little

COLD? You don't see me crying about MY C-disease, do you? Smile! Everything will be OK."

Without missing a beat, Joe, who was driving, turned to me and said, "Seriously, Mom? We're a little tired of hearing about your chlamydia already."

He and I burst into laughter, and even Rachel grinned for a split second. I couldn't see Adam's reaction but hope he was smiling, too. In that moment, I knew that my kids and our laughter would be my first line of defense in getting through the months to come. (No offense to anyone who has had chlamydia as I'm certain it's no laughing matter, but you have to admit, when a son accuses his 50-something mom of having an STD, it's a pretty humorous moment.)

And so, I committed to observing every detail of the adventure ahead, if for no other reason than to see if I could uncover some humor. I've always believed that when we're laughing, we're living, and at this particularly pivotal moment in time, I knew unequivocally that I wanted to live.

Think about it. Would you rather laugh your way through cancer or let your chin drag on the floor? Not only is laughing great for you physically, but it can also pump up your courage as you head into doctor appointments, biopsies, scans — even surgery and chemo. It's tough to find the energy to fret and freak out when you're busy seeking out the silly and absurd.

The gift of cancer — no, really. OK, so maybe I'm really pressing it now with the Pollyanna attitude, but hear me out. I know this diagnosis can be devastating and the experience is never an easy one, but look at your cancer from another angle for a minute — as an opportunity and a gift. Few circumstances in life will bring you closer to the people around you and to your own spiritual center. Cancer helps us rediscover, or maybe discover for the first time, the boundless strength of our own souls, and the kindness, generosity, and selflessness of the people around us. In some magical stroke of irony, one of the most loathsome diseases of our time brings people together to rally for a common cause. Suddenly we realize that politics, religion, age, and other issues that far too often keep us at arm's length from one another no longer apply.

In this way, breast cancer became the most empowering and enlightening experience of my life. I'm a different person today — stronger, happier, and whole in a way I simply was not before. My wish for you is that you feel this empowerment, too.

Why I ultimately picked up my pen. As breast cancer goes, I guess I had a pretty decent case of it. Ductal with a big old tumor in the left, lobular scattered throughout the right, and malignant lymph nodes on both sides. This diagnosis meant I got the full breadth of experiences: surgery, chemo, radiation, drugs, complications, and, of course, the emotional ups and downs inherent in a situation where biopsy results and treatment side effects become your everyday routine.

But I was blessed in having not only a wonderful family to stand beside me, but also a friend and breast cancer mentor who held my hand and showed me the way, steeling me for the difficult moments and joining me in celebration of the good ones. My longtime pal Mary Jane had been diagnosed several years earlier, and her courage, drive, and never-ending optimism in the face of metastatic breast cancer helped me see the true power of inner strength and faith. As she continues to live her life full to the brim with love and joy, MJ truly is one of those heroes people talk about. With her at my side as cancer coach extraordinaire, I felt invincible.

Every person diagnosed with cancer should have this sense of security, I thought. Everyone should have a friend or mentor who has walked the path before. I found, unfortunately, that this wasn't the case.

My friend Andrea, for example, whom I met in the radiation waiting room (I would have my treatment each morning and then pass the baton to her), told me that when she was diagnosed, she had no point of reference for navigating all that was about to happen to her. No one close to her had experienced cancer. That was a very different perspective from my own, since I had watched both of my parents overcome cancer. Over many years, my dad went through several surgeries, as well as chemotherapy and radiation treatments, to beat colon cancer, and my mom pushed a rare form of lymphoma into remission through a clinical trial that had been her only hope of survival. Add Mary Jane into that mix, and I knew almost by osmosis how to cope with cancer; I had learned from the best. But Andrea had no mentors or coaches. Throughout her journey, she wished for someone who could help her navigate — a "bosom buddy" who could offer coping tools, candor, and camaraderie.

Hearing Andrea's story helped me see that chronicling my adventures with cancer might be helpful to others. So I took notes. Now I'm sharing them with you, hoping they might help you navigate your *own* journey; understand, accept, and honor your feelings; and, most of all, reassure you that you are never, ever alone in this. If you start to feel alone at any point, remind yourself that you are surrounded by *many* people who have overcome this challenge before you, who are facing it along with you, or who have found a way to incorporate it into their day-to-day reality. None of us asked to be part of this club, but we're in it together just the same. My advice: Embrace the humorous moments. Soak in the love of the people who support you. Face every hurdle with faith and resolve. And above all, believe in the innate strength of your soul.

THE JOURNEY BEGINS

FlatTop

Chapter 1
I Have *WHAT?*

If your journey starts out a little rugged, don't despair.

Hearing the news you have cancer is a moment like no other. We hear of people overcoming cancer every day, but somehow this doesn't lessen the impact of hearing the diagnosis ourselves. Maybe that's because we've all also heard stories of people — or lived through experiences with loved ones — where the outcome wasn't as positive.

So when we get that diagnosis, maybe we think about death for a moment. Maybe we wonder if this diagnosis means that we're running out of time. Maybe we slip into a fight-or-flight response wishing we could turn the clock back to when we didn't have cancer — or, at least, when we didn't *know* we had it. Man, those were the days, huh?

But then something incredible happens. It may take as little as a few minutes, or as long as days or months. In a single moment of clarity that holds the power to carry us through our entire cancer experience, we realize that we're much stronger than we thought. We become grateful that it is us, rather than someone close to us, who is facing this disease. *What if it were my daughter or son, my sister or brother, my mom or dad, my nephew or niece? Thank God it is me, because I know in my heart that I can handle this.* In this moment, fear is replaced with confidence, resolve, and reassuring self-love. This is the moment we all need to recognize and embrace.

But I'm getting ahead of myself. Let's go back to the moment of diagnosis. What was yours like? As all of these thoughts and feelings — or maybe it was numbness — swirled around you, what was your doctor saying and doing? Did you get the news in a supportive, positive manner? Or was the experience less than ideal? If it was the latter, do *not* despair. I have heard plenty of stories from plenty of women who would have scripted this life-changing moment much differently, yet their long-term journey turned out just fine.

They're not coming back OK. Following my mammogram, follow-up mammogram and ultrasound, I was told I had a "mass" in my left breast and some "suspicious calcifications" in the right. All would require biopsies. I was referred to a surgeon for a preliminary examination before these tests would ensue. As I lay on the table with this seasoned surgeon feeling around and asking questions, I asked *her* one: "If the biopsies come back OK, will you still want to remove the mass?"

She looked at me as if I had missed the whole story line and scoffed, "They're not coming back OK."

I went numb and had no idea what to do next. Assume the fetal position? Cover my ears and sing "La, la, la, la — can't hear you" very loudly? Shriek? For a moment I pictured myself taking her face in both of my hands, pulling it within an inch of my own and demanding through gritted teeth, "What did you just say? No. What. Did. You. Just. SAY?" Instead, I remained stoically silent as she finished her exam and cavalierly instructed me to go across the hall for biopsies. Really? This was how I was introduced to the concept of having cancer? This is how my life turned in a single moment from being someone who did not have cancer to someone who did?

Having needles plunged into my breasts sounded like as good a way as any to celebrate this news.

You're a 12. Andrea had quite a diagnostic experience, too. She had gone for a mammogram to rule out breast cancer as her doctor tried to identify the root cause of some unusual swelling she had been experiencing. After her test, the medical practitioner summoned her into an office and asked if it would be OK for the hospital's two interns to sit in on the conversation. "We're trying to give them the opportunity to experience the whole range of possible situations," she explained.

Red flag, Andrea, red flag! Slightly anxious and completely confused, Andrea nodded slowly.

The medical practitioner continued, "You have breast cancer. And on a scale from 1 to 10, with 1 being we're not very concerned and 10 being we're extremely concerned, your situation is a 12."

Freight train 1, Andrea 0. *This* was the best approach they could come up with? (What. We *told* her to sit down, didn't we?)

Back up, dude! One more: My cousin Judy went for a follow-up mammogram and sonogram when the results from her routine test had come back with "something suspicious." Midway through the ultrasound procedure, the attending doctor, who had been viewing the test from behind a wall, burst into the room, his panic-stricken face coming to rest just inches from Judy's.

"I am 99.9 percent certain this is cancer. You must have a biopsy NOW!" he demanded. Judy was, understandably, taken aback. When she didn't immediately respond, the doctor repeated — faster, more closely, and more loudly this time, "I am 99.9 percent certain this is cancer. You must have a biopsy NOW!"

Instinctively, Judy held both hands up, palms outward in front of her face, and said, "Dude, back UP!"

The doctor froze, stared, and then turned and walked away in silence. "You've offended him," the technician said, shaking her head.

OH! *I've* offended *HIM?* Well, by all means go make sure he's OK, Judy thought to herself as she made her way to the dressing room to reclaim her clothes. There would be no biopsy under this doctor's care.

Just a thought. I'm not one to be overly critical of others, and I have the deepest respect for those who selflessly practice medicine, but I've been thinking that maybe some of them could benefit from sensitivity training of some sort: maybe a course called "Empathy: How to Deliver a Frightening Diagnosis." You know, when I was a kid, I watched a lot of movies where they would call patients in for a special appointment when test results came back with less than inspiring results. Sure, the patients had an inkling that something was up, but at least they had a chance to ease into the situation rather than being blindsided. They also had the opportunity to invite a family member to come along and sit beside them, at the ready with hugs and reassurance.

Could doctors do this today? *Do* some of them still do this? I'm certain the answer is yes on both counts. My doctor didn't, though. Nor did many of my friends' doctors. But hey: Maybe it's not their social skills that should be called into question. Maybe it's just the way we live today, in hyperspeed, expecting instant gratification on every front, including that straight-shooting diagnosis that sometimes can be more of a hypothesis than a proven statement of fact. (We always have to wait for biopsy results to get the whole story anyway, so why not wait to tell us when you're 100-percent certain?) It's likely that at least part of the issue is related to how we overwork our doctors. They simply don't have time to give every patient coddling time. So unfortunately, possibly more often than not, we are presented with a matter-of-fact, don't-you-dare-act-like-a-baby-and-cry-about-this attitude. "They're not coming back OK. Put your big-girl pants on, deal with it, and scoot on over to get those biopsies stat. We're on a schedule here, you know."

What's the point? My point is that your journey may start out a little rugged. In fact, whether your diagnosis is delivered with no empathy at all or all the empathy in the world, you might lose your balance or your cool for a bit. That's perfectly natural. But once you regain your footing, there are things you can do every day going forward to make your experience better. So don't dwell on the diagnosis. Dig right in to get to the solutions. Get yourself moving forward in a positive direction and keep that positive momentum going. A good starting point is to take steps to build a great medical team to support you.

Chapter 2
Who's With Me?

You deserve a doc who looks this disease in the eye every day and says, "Not on my watch."

I would never suggest that you ditch a doctor just because the diagnosis experience was disappointing. But do trust your gut if you're getting more explicit warning signs that this might not be a good fit for you. I gave my diagnosing surgeon another chance, another visit, before deciding to find someone else. I asked my sister, Debbie, to come along, because I value her personal and medical opinions (she works in the biz). After spending five minutes with this doctor, Deb's vote was to cut and run. I knew she was right. The doc and I just didn't have chemistry. I wondered if she could have chemistry with *anyone*, based on her callous attitude, probably developed over years of having to deliver unwanted diagnoses. While I was sympathetic to her life experience, I didn't feel that this was the right time for me to compromise on what I wanted: a doctor I could talk to, who would listen and care, and who instinctively knew the best course of action for my circumstances.

I found that doctor when a friend shared his wife's experience. Her surgeon had worked something of a miracle after she'd been told by another doc that her prognosis was extremely negative. Today, years later, she is healthy, happy, and grateful. This was the kind of ending I wanted to my own story, so I made an appointment with this surgeon. Turns out he is one of the world's kindest, warmest, and most competent surgeons in his field. Once he had done his part, the bilateral mastectomy, he recommended the world's kindest, warmest, most competent oncologist. How lucky was I?

I can't express the importance of holding out for the right doctors. Depending on your circumstances, you may need a whole slew of them — specialists in surgery, oncology, radiation, and possibly plastic surgery, cardiology, or other areas of expertise. Maybe you can't interview every one of them before allowing them to become involved in your treatment program, but do what you can. Get recommendations from people you trust: your family doctor, OB/GYN, friends who have had breast cancer — heck, I even asked my pharmacist. This is not a time for inviting just anyone to join the party. Find out what people are saying, what kind of results they've achieved, and remember that you deserve the best.

How do you know when you've gotten the best? When you're comfortable letting your doctor see you naked. I don't mean bodily naked; that goes without saying. I'm talking about seeing your naked soul. You need to feel that you can open up to ask every question, and share your concerns and fears with this person. If they're the right doctor for you, then they will hear you. They'll address any issue you want to discuss and be straightforward about your options. As you make the choices that you inevitably must make, they will support you with every tool in their bag.

My oncologist *is* this extraordinary person. From the day we met, Dr. Lois has been in my court. She gave me the lowdown on my situation, told me what to expect from the treatment, and watched me like a hawk to make sure I was holding up. When the standard chemo protocol became too much for my body, she brainstormed alternate solutions that still got the good poison into me but in a kinder, gentler fashion. When I expressed concerns about my symptoms and conditions, she offered encouragement. Even today, as I see her for follow-up visits to ensure my ongoing health, she always has a new study to tell me about and new ideas for keeping me — and all of us in the BC lifeboat — alive and well.

I like to think that if she weren't my oncologist, Dr. Lois would still be my friend. Because aside from being the best freaking oncologist on the planet, she is one of the bravest and most caring human beings I have had the honor to meet. Think about this: You and I somehow wandered into cancer's path. But Dr. Lois and her ilk — wonderful, selfless, committed doctors — CHOOSE cancer. They choose to look this disease in the face every day and say, "Not on my watch." The best of these doctors hold our hands when we're too weak to hold up our own heads, navigate new courses when the tests aren't coming up quite as we'd like, and understand that not a single one of us is a "case" or a statistic.

Here's an example of what I'm talking about: When my chemotherapy and radiation treatments ended, Dr. Lois explained that my port should stay in for at least a year or two, just in case I should need further treatment. Recurrence would most likely happen in the first few years, she said, and most women like to keep the port in so that they won't need another surgery to install a new one if that need arises. I explained why that didn't work for me.

"It has to go," I told her. "You may not be able to prove it, but I know in my heart that I'm healed, and this [tapping the port lightly] feels too much like an invitation for cancer to come back. I need to be free of it." Without hesitation, she smiled and said, "Out it comes then."

See why I love her?

Find your Dr. Lois. Trust me. Having the right doctor — the one who gets where you're coming from and guides your path ahead — makes all the difference.

FlatTop

Chapter 3
You Are NOT a Statistic

What's true for someone else may not be true for you.

I just mentioned how important it is for doctors to understand that we aren't statistics, but we have to understand this, too, and live our lives accordingly. Listen and believe: You are *not* a statistic. You are an individual, and your future health depends on *your* experience and *your* attitude — not anyone else's and not any group's.

During the follow-up visit with my surgeon, he explained that both of the two lymph nodes they took from my right side were malignant. On the left, it was two out of 16. "Could have been worse, huh?" I said, hoping to reassure us both.

He wasn't quite as enthusiastic about this outcome as I was. "I guess you could look at it that way," he said politely. "But, honestly, it's not the scenario we were hoping for. We're going to need to be aggressive with chemotherapy and radiation."

When I went home, I started looking at statistics — outcomes, lifespan, and such. As I scanned the "Stage 3, 4+ Nodes" columns, I started to see what he was talking about and spent several sobering moments allowing my brain to soak in the data. Then, as if snapping out of a hypnotic trance, I physically shook those numbers out of my head, grinned, and said, *Screw that,* to no one in particular. *I'm not a statistic. I don't have to play by these rules.*

I looked over at Cancer Bear, my first official cancer gift, who became a source of comfort throughout my journey (thanks to my pal Jodi, who understands that we are *never* too old for a bear hug). As he sat on my nightstand, I imagined CB winking and giving me the thumbs-up (well, the paws-up, I suppose, since opposable thumbs aren't really his strong suit). Then I thought of my mother's admonition when I was in grade school: *If everyone jumped off a bridge, would you jump off the bridge just to be like them? No, Mom,* I'd say reluctantly, rolling my eyes and sulking in the corner because I secretly wished I *could* be like everyone else, bridge or otherwise. But not today. Today I was going to set my own course for the future.

Thanks, Mom. You, too, Cancer Bear.

I can tell you this with certainty: Facts about what has happened to others in your situation are irrelevant. You are unique — designed differently from anyone else and charged with your own brand of pluck and determination. So don't waste your time looking at lists of numbers that simply don't apply to you. Set your own course and stick with it!

That goes for *words* on the web, too — not just numbers! There will inevitably be times when you will need or want more information about this condition, that drug, or an upcoming procedure. Try to get as much information as you can from your doctor or other members of your medical team you really trust. If you feel like you need to tap the internet for more information, use only reliable, objective, bona fide medical sources and take comments from patients with a grain of salt.

Here's why. People who sail through a course of treatment smoothly seldom think to go online and share their story. Most often, it's those who have negative experiences who want to vent or send out a warning to others. The problem with this is that what harms one person can be the ticket to healing for another. Someone else's details about their dramatic reaction to a certain drug or treatment might discourage you from trying it when, in fact, it may affect you in a completely different way.

I had read horror stories online about a certain drug that was to be part of my treatment plan. Some women said that the pain caused by this marrow stimulant was unbearable. I asked my oncologist if I could forgo it. No. It was an important part of the protocol, she said. So I tried it. And guess what? Zero pain. Had I insisted on moving forward without this drug, I would not have been able to tolerate my chemo. Taking this a step further, I probably would not be here today to write this book.

Bottom line: Your body is different from mine, your neighbor's, and your sister's. You shouldn't make judgments based on other people's experiences. Don't even read those horror stories on the internet. They serve no helpful purpose.

Having said that, it *is* important that you build your knowledge about your disease and treatment protocol. You need to be able to understand what your doctors are telling you and advocate on your own behalf when you believe something doesn't quite fit your circumstances. So seek information; just be discerning. Make sure the source is reputable and unbiased.

You'll also find that there are some great online communities where people with breast cancer support one another. If you're inclined to join one and it brings you comfort, enjoy the camaraderie! But remember that even friends who are close to you can have very different experiences. You are one of a kind!

Chapter 4
Letting People In

Why go it alone?

From the start, doctors and nurses described cancer to me as a "family disease," and they were right on the money. They weren't referring to heredity (even though, of course, heredity can play a role); rather, they were talking about how cancer reaches far beyond our own bodies to torment the people who love us. While we bear the physical brunt of the disease, the emotional toll it takes on our families and friends can be just as great — sometimes, far greater.

Your family undoubtedly believes in your strength, courage, and resolve, but it's just human nature to worry and want to help. Family members and close friends too often feel like bystanders — like no matter what they do, it won't be enough. They want some measure of control, to stop you from hurting, to remove that possibility that they might lose you, and to save you from the rigors of surgery, treatment, and recovery that may lie ahead. Unfortunately, that control is out of reach. And so the people who love you feel completely helpless.

I was personally hit over the head with this reality shortly after recovering from cancer myself. There I was, celebrating life, soaring on the high of my reentry into good health, when cancer knocked again. Only this time, it brought me to my knees. Because this time, it wasn't *my* cancer. It was my sister's.

Like our entire family, I was blindsided. What were the odds that Debbie, my constant companion since the day I opened my eyes to see her peering over the edge of my bassinet, would be stricken with the same disease I had faced just a couple of years before? I had illogically concluded that I had taken one for the team on this — that somehow Deb would be safe because I had fulfilled our obligation on the breast cancer front. How *dare* cancer come back for another piece of us, I thought. How dare it challenge us again. Hadn't we passed the test? Mom, Dad, me — we'd all been pretty darned good sports about the whole cancer thing. Now Deb had to weather it, too? She had just finished holding my hand through all of *my* ups and downs. Why should she have to go through all of that *again?* I was indignant.

My response to her diagnosis reminded me of the sinking feeling I had experienced when my dad, and later my mom, had been diagnosed. There was not the sense of empowerment I felt with my own diagnosis but rather an overwhelming sense of helplessness. And yes, I fully recognize the flip-flop in my attitude. The positivity and spirituality that had permeated every corner of my own cancer experience was suddenly absent when it came to my sister's diagnosis. I was, in a word, *pissed.* And it took some doing — a lot of deep meditation and prayer — to overcome these negative feelings and get back to a spiritual balance that would enable me to offer Deb the positive support she needed. That's the power this disease wields over us when it strikes someone we love. It pulls the rug right out from under us.

This is why your loved ones need you as much as you need them right now. You will take care of one another dealing with this family disease. From your perspective, that means letting them in. Talking with them. Sharing your experience and feelings. Letting them do things for you and helping them understand that even the tiniest actions can bring you comfort. Helping them see that just having them with you is the best medicine you could possibly ask for. Above all, including them in every tiny victory you achieve along the way.

One of the most beautiful things about cancer is that it has the potential to bring us closer to the people we love than we may have ever been before. It helps us recognize and reach into the depths of our individual and collective strengths, and move forward together toward a common goal. When you let your loved ones in, you will awaken the most positive emotions you can imagine and build upon one another's strengths by facing the path ahead united.

If you don't have family or friends close by (or even if you do), watch for opportunities to make friends along your way. Where cancer lives, hearts (your own and others') open wider than ever before. In just a bit, I'll talk about pulling those others into the fold, but first, I'll address family issues.

Telling your family. Unless your family is in the room with you when you hear your diagnosis for the first time, you'll face the dubious task of telling them the news. You know it's going to be hard on them, because it was hard on you when you heard it, wasn't it? But it has to be done, so steel yourself, take a deep breath, and just do it.

You probably know whom this news will hit hardest: your spouse, kids, parents, brother, sister, best friend — you just know who it'll be. For me, it was my kids. Of course, I knew my parents and siblings would feel the pain, too, but they had been through cancer and other diseases with loved ones before. I knew they'd be OK. But my kids? Man. The thought of telling them ripped my heart right out of my chest.

As a parent, your instinct is to protect your kids from pain, no matter how old they are or how much you recognize and respect their emotional strength. Although I was fully prepared to face the circumstances myself, I could not bring myself to break the news. I concocted a delusional plan to keep it from them until I had made it through the rough parts. All three of them were away at school, so I figured I could put on a good face when they came home for weekends and spare them the day-to-day details of what I'd be going through.

"You're not thinking straight, honey," Deb said in the comforting big-sister tone that I always recognize as her way of gently reprimanding me when she really wants to say, "Have you lost your freaking *mind*?" I had told her about my diagnosis first so that she could help me navigate next steps at a time when I felt somewhat lost. From the time we were kids, I've relied on Deb as my confidante and compass, so it was only natural I'd lean on her for advice on how to tell the rest of the family. "Not telling them wouldn't be fair to them," she continued. "They'll want to be with you in surgery and to help you recuperate. Let them be part of this."

My pal Brad, who has a gift for seeing matters pragmatically, wasn't nearly as diplomatic. "Yeah, you've lost your freaking mind," he confirmed. "What if something happens during surgery? They'll never forgive you. They deserve to know. You've gotta tell them now."

Well, of course they were right, and I was grateful that they helped me see things more clearly. I was just being a big, fat chicken. So, after playing the scenario over in my head a thousand times to calculate how to hurt them the least, I took that deep breath and made the very difficult words move from my brain to my mouth.

It was the hardest conversation I have ever had, with any*one* about any*thing*. I told them over a dinner I had prepared at home, speaking as matter-of-factly as possible, and offering technical details that, at the time, pointed to a very positive outcome. I assured them I was up to the challenge and that they shouldn't worry. In spite of this promise, I watched shock take over the three of them, as surely as if they had been struck by lightning. My psyche went into autopilot and I blurted out a take on one of the boys' favorite stupid jokes: "So when the doctor told me, guess what I said? I said, 'CANCER? I hardly know her!'"

They didn't think that was funny at all. I mean, Joe high-fived me, but it was an auto-pilot move, and that positive clap instantly gave way to an awkward, deafening silence around the table.

It's definitely not an easy conversation, but once you get through it, it paves the way for you to face the road ahead … together.

Your family deserves to know why you're tired. Or nauseated. Or out of touch. (Yes, it will be noticeable.) They will want to help, and that's a good thing — good for them, and good for you. Of course, you need to keep in mind the age of your children. Their need-to-know level will differ depending on their maturity level. If they're very young, you might be able to get away with "Mommy's not feeling well," or something similar. One of my friends told me that had been best for her elementary-age children. Beyond "very young," though, explain as much as you feel you can so that they understand what to expect as you go through surgery, treatment, and recuperation. Few things are as frightening to children *or* adults as the unknown.

As for my children, they grew stronger that night and in the months to come, as they realized that the person who had held them for so many years suddenly needed to *be* held. To my endless pride, they rose to the occasion and then some:

Rachel became nothing short of my private nurse. She changed her schedule at school so she could alternate with Deb in driving me to, and holding my hand at, oncology appointments and chemo treatments. She made food for me and encouraged me to eat on those days when eating was the last thing on my mind. And she kept running lists of my side effects and symptoms to share with my doctors. Rachel's ability to gauge my physical and psychological strength at any moment was uncanny, and, to my delight, she never tired of belting out one more chorus of "Radioactive" with me while we watched those IV fluids drip.

Joe offered his own brand of support, taking care of the yardwork and things around the house, telling me funny stories to keep my spirits high, and reassuring me about things like my baldness. "C'mon, Mom," he teased, "let's see what you look like bald. Take off your scarf." To my surprise, when I did, he didn't flinch, scream, or laugh. Instead, he said, "You are rockin' it, Mom. I'm so serious. Why do you cover it up? You should have shaved your head a long time ago." Hm. Why hadn't *I* thought of that?

Adam stood strong and ready to jump in anytime I needed help. Although he, like Rachel and Joe, was away at school, it seemed he always happened to be home for my worst moments — the Saturday morning he took me to the ER for IV fluids, the day he sat beside me,

31

reassuring me when my memory seemed to abandon me completely, and the painfully emotional afternoon of my final chemo treatment, when he offered comforting support after I confessed that I couldn't physically withstand that one last hit.

The moral of this story? While it may be excruciating to tell them about it, your disease has the potential to bring out the superstars in your children. Think about what you can teach them through this experience, too. You can show them through your own behavior how to navigate rough waters, how to believe in themselves no matter how difficult life becomes, and how to hold onto their faith and never let go.

Telling friends and colleagues. Sometimes people (looking at you, Rachel!) tell me I'm too trusting of others. I think that's impossible. Given half a chance, people are awesome, especially in circumstances like this. Yet some of us choose to "protect" ourselves from others when we have cancer. We're silent about our situation at a time when we really could use some support because, after all, what will people think? Will they view us as weak?

Incompetent? Pathetic? Will they turn their backs on us because they don't know what to say or how to act around us? Will they stop joking around with us because they think we're dying?

From experience, I'll say "probably not" to all of these. I believe that openness is the best policy. That's not to say you should blurt out "I have cancer!" in the middle of the grocery store, but for the people already in your world, doesn't it make sense to let them know you're going through a rough time? Maybe they'll pray for you. Maybe they have experience with cancer and can offer you some valuable advice. Or maybe they will just appreciate that you trusted them enough to let them see your vulnerability, and it will strengthen your relationship with them forever.

I know that sometimes people aren't comfortable talking with you personally when you have cancer. They'll send cards, flowers, gifts, and prayers, but there's something about cancer that makes some people uneasy about being face-to-face or even talking on the phone. Maybe it's because cancer still has that death stigma attached to it. I don't know. But don't hold it against them.

Whether they speak to you or say a silent prayer, they're with you, and that's what really matters.

A friend of mine refrained from telling others about her cancer because, as a business owner, she feared that her clients wouldn't trust her with their accounts anymore. A business owner myself, I found the opposite to be true. Clients offered me just as many, if not more, projects as I went through my hospitalizations and treatments. They were also very understanding on the occasions when I had to say no. So when I needed to be in bed resting, I could be in bed resting. My friend, on the other hand, had to work through some very difficult days. She would have been so much better off had she been able to take days off here and there, instead of pushing herself to work because people expected her to be as productive as she'd always been.

Which brings me right back to the statement that people are awesome. Give them a chance. Let them in!

Welcome new friends, too. Throughout my life, I've felt very lucky to have wonderful friends. Dating back to first grade, when I first realized that strangers could magically turn into friends, I've held a sacred appreciation for those who so openly offer love and support to others.

I was, you see, the kid who threw up in the class coat closet every morning. Of course I didn't mean to. In fact, each day when I woke up, I would tell my 5-year-old self that this would be the day I'd make it through the morning vomit-free. But the smell of the endless sea of plastic lunchboxes, wafting through the air on the school bus and then in the classroom, said otherwise. Inevitably, I would foul the neatly arranged row of rubber over-the-shoe pull-on boots with the contents of my anxiety-ridden belly.

Some people — my teacher, the janitor, and many of my classmates — were not kind. And who could blame them? I wouldn't want to pull my boot on and feel that particular brand of squish, nor be the person responsible for sprinkling that oatmeal-looking sawdust onto the mess prior to sweeping it up and carting it off to wherever recovered schoolchild vomit goes.

Still, I wished that I didn't have to spend the better part of every school day cowering in shame, shrinking from the inevitable, relentless taunting and wishing I could be anywhere but there. I felt alone. Vulnerable. Scared.

Then something remarkable happened. Margaret sat with me at lunch. Betty offered to lend me her thick red pencil when I lost my own. And Susan asked if I wanted to play together at recess. These kindnesses, in the face of my severe grossness, formed the foundation of my learning to trust people outside of my own family. I always knew my family had my back, because, well, that was mandatory, right? But I recognized that by extending their friendship to the closet puker, these brave young girls were laying their own reputations on the line. I learned from my worst childhood experience one of my best life lessons: When we open our hearts, wonderful people step forward to fill them.

And so, when you share the news that you have cancer, remember that it's not just old friends who will support you, but new ones, too. Strangers may become friends and some of the fiercest advocates you've ever had (yes, even if you throw up chemo juice in their boots).

I met so many warm, kind, wonderful people — not only in medical settings, where we spend so much of our time, but also out in the world at large. A stranger approached me in the grocery store one day, placing her hand supportively on my arm as I guided my shopping cart, and simply said, "I was where you are just a couple of years ago. Don't lose hope and don't give up. If I could do it, YOU can do it!" Aside from dashing my fantasy that my headscarf might have looked like a fashion statement, this stranger-turned-friend (if only for a moment) was a very influential voice in my head whenever the going got tough.

I would imagine that group support sessions or survivor workshops would be a great source of new friends. In hindsight, I regret that I didn't become involved in any of these. I did, however, meet plenty of people in waiting rooms, infusion rooms, hospital hallways, and other venues where I had never expected to be. What I found was that people tend to be very open and kind when they're in the throes of cancer. There's an understanding among our group that transcends geography, social class, politics, and even interests. No one's in a hurry like we all seem to be when we're healthy — too busy to talk, places to go, people to see, you know. Cancer stops us in our tracks and reminds us that every person we meet is important, and every conversation dear.

We see people differently. We see their grace. Their beauty. Their uniqueness. And so we reach out to one another, talking, sharing insights, and trying to make the path even slightly better for them as they take the next step forward. I have had some of the most genuine conversations of my life with people I knew for only five or 10 minutes.

Once you've met these kindred spirits, you're likely to wonder why you were ever uncomfortable around people with cancer. Before I went through cancer myself, I didn't really know how to talk to people who had it. Like so many others, I would feel awkward and worry I'd say the wrong thing, have the wrong look on my face, or, Heaven forbid, let them see me cry for them. Now when I hear someone has cancer, I want to meet them, talk with them, laugh and cry with them right out loud, and squeeze their hand to let them know that no matter how rough things might get, they are never alone.

Since I've come out on the other side of cancer, my friends introduce me to friends who are going through cancers of all kinds. I welcome these visits with all my heart. One very special woman was nearing the end of her brief journey with pancreatic cancer when I met her. She struggled with pain, uncertainty, and the speed at which the disease was progressing. Although I hadn't experienced anything close to the extent of the disease that she had, I was completely comfortable talking with her about whatever was on her mind: living, dying, hurting, healing, hoping, coping.

These conversations are necessary and precious. And when we share this sacred bond, it becomes a lifelong gift. Our "cancer friends" help strengthen and sustain us, and we strengthen and sustain them right back. Throughout your life, this kindred link will connect you with people whose beauty and kindness you might otherwise have missed.

And so, keep the phrase "the more, the merrier" in mind. Let people in. All of them. There's no need to go this alone. Why would anyone ever want to?

Chapter 5
Embracing Spiritual Strength

When our bodies are at their weakest, our souls have the potential to become their strongest.

No matter how positive our attitudes might be, and how open we are to laughing at some of the situations that come our way, there is obviously a very sobering side to our cancer experience. Regardless of our diagnosis or prognosis, cancer tests our spirit by pushing us to explore our own mortality. This exploration can be peaceful and comforting or downright frightening, depending on how we choose to engage ourselves and our beliefs.

I realize, of course, that your beliefs are likely different from mine, in one way or a thousand ways, but we all believe *something*. It's that something I'm referring to when I use the terms "spirituality" and "faith." Spirituality could be your religion, your connection to the universal life force, or your belief in your own intrinsic power, while faith is your commitment to that religion, connection, or belief. "Spirituality" and "faith" are simply my shorthand for talking about what or whom we tap into for guidance with challenges, moral decisions, and everyday living.

When you were diagnosed, what did you do — cry? deny? ask *Why?* Or did you take a deep breath and assure yourself that spiritual strength would be surrounding you, holding your hand and picking you up anytime you might fall?

Each of us reacts differently and, to my knowledge, no initial response is better than another. But to truly come out of this experience whole and at peace, I believe that we need to move beyond the negativity of crying, stamping our feet, denying reality, or succumbing to sadness to ultimately arrive at the latter option, where we accept our situation and know in the depth of our souls that unconditional love is with us. At the point when we recognize and embrace the spiritual strength that comes from within and perhaps from the wider universe, we learn one of the greatest lessons of life: We are never given a heavier burden than we can bear. Sometimes we just underestimate ourselves. In the right frame of mind, open to the spiritual strength that's available to each of us, we actually do have the potential to become superhuman.

One of my Christian friends shared this passage with me: "If God brings you *to* it, He will lead you *through* it." In other words, if those test results come back saying things you don't like, it doesn't mean you've been abandoned. In fact, the opposite is true. Just keep believing, holding your faith close and knowing that, as you're doing the sometimes difficult work of healing, you are never alone.

Patience is critical, too. My cousin Linda, who faced her own breast cancer with unshakable strength and resolve, continues to reassure me that, no matter how long it takes for our prayers to be answered, God is always listening. "Sometimes it's difficult to trust in God's perfect timing, but we must; He hears every prayer," she says. "In the moment, it can be hard to wrap our heads around the lessons we're meant to learn from all of this, but they're in there somewhere. If we don't see them on this side of

Heaven, we will surely see them on the other. Until then, we need to just keep loving and helping one another."

Your powerful, soaring spirit. Before cancer, I thought my faith was strong. But I had no idea how much deeper it could become. If you've already experienced this yourself, then you know what I'm talking about. If not, then maybe my experience will be helpful to you.

The best way I can explain this is to say that where before I BELIEVED, today I KNOW. Through this gift of disease comes the potential for enlightenment that turns your faith, belief, and hope into a *knowing* that becomes etched into your soul. You come to understand with great certainty that you have the strength to go wherever your journey might take you — that with universal love and spirituality, you have absolutely got this!

I woke up to this knowledge when my body was at its weakest, while I was deep into chemo. As I was flattened into my mattress, overcome with nausea and fatigue, and with anemia shortening my breath, I felt a comforting presence lift me up and reassure me that all was well. I was certain that God had sent angels and family members who had passed to watch over me. But it was even more than that: As I looked around at the handmade blankets, handwritten notes, healing stones, flowers, and other gifts from friends and family, I could feel their loving presence, too, supporting me as if they were sitting right next to my bed, holding my hand. In these moments, my spirit transcended physical strife and knew without a hint of doubt that I was absolutely safe and unconditionally loved. There was no sense of fear or danger. Only peace.

And although my personal introduction to the limitlessness of spirit came about during a period of physical incapacitation, I don't believe that is a prerequisite for feeling this pure, encompassing love. You might never feel this low physically. I hope you don't! Just know that, regardless of your physical state, you can tap into this loving force any day at any time simply by being present in the moment and opening your heart. When you're open, the loving spirit of the universe will never let go of your hand. Everyone who loves you, whether they are physically next to you or not, can be right there with you.

Deeper, more meaningful connections. When you get to this *knowing* place, you'll begin to develop greater vision. When you look into the faces of those around you — family, friends, and strangers alike — it will be as if all of the packaging has been stripped away and you're looking straight into the essence of every beautiful soul. As people generously reach out to you, your spiritual circle will become complete. It won't be just *you* looking into cancer's eyes anymore; it will be every person and spirit who supports you.

It occurred to me more than once that this is how we should live every day. In this moment of unity, life takes on clarity that most of us simply don't have access to when we're well, caught up in the hectic pace of our physical world, where we seem to slip into a day-to-day-grind mentality that sucks the energy from our souls. What if we stopped talking so much and instead really listened? If we quit crying about the things that trouble us and instead rejoice in what is good, true, and sustaining?

Chapter 6
Give Yourself a Break!

If you don't like to swear, then cancer probably isn't the disease for you.

Before we get into the rough stuff — surgery, chemo, and radiation — let's regroup on the topic of being positive. Is it important to stay positive? Yes. Is it possible to be positive 100 percent of the time? Mmmmmm, probably not.

I mean, maybe we find the strength to be optimistic 70, 80, 90 percent of the time (maybe 95 if you have a good supply of chocolate), but give yourself a break now and then. No matter how much of an overachiever you might be, don't expect yourself to be 100 percent strong or 100 percent positive every minute of every day. We're all human!

I can't tell you how many times I would see things that needed to be done — dishes that needed to be washed, work projects that needed attention — and wish I had the energy and presence of mind to do them, but I simply didn't. Sometimes that made me cry. *Who can't walk over to the sink and wash a glass?* I'd think, frustrated by the immobilization I'd often feel during treatment.

One of the worst of these moments happened a few days after a particularly difficult chemo session, when I stood at the bottom of my staircase contemplating whether peeing my pants was a preferable solution to climbing those daunting eight stairs to the bathroom. I ended up crawling up on my hands and knees, cursing cancer every step of the way. *They should see me now,* I thought sardonically of the people who regularly praised me for what they perceived to be insuperable optimism.

They weren't entirely wrong, though. These definitely were outlying moments, but looking back, I'm certain that allowing myself to occasionally let off some steam through tears, anger, and the all-powerful swear was good. Even when we see cancer as the precious gift it can be, and even if we're able to visualize ourselves in the healthy, thriving bodies we intend to be sometime very soon, there's no shame in giving in to our own humanity once in a while. So if you need to cry now and then; if you need to ask someone to come with you to a doctor's appointment for no reason other than you just can't face it alone today; if you ever feel yourself going to a weaker place for whatever reason, it's OK. In fact, it's more than OK: It's natural! I would worry more about you if you never had these moments. Just try not to stay in that place too long. Remember that this low feeling is temporary, and that you have the resilience to come back to positive no matter how many times you may drift into the negative.

About that swearing. Ah, sweet relief. I admit that I was no stranger to cursing before my diagnosis. Growing up, I saw how well it worked for my dad when he missed the nail and hammered his thumb instead. (I would picture the cartoon symbols all around him, like in the Sunday comics.) So I tried the swear myself when I was 10 or 11. Of course, I only muttered it under my breath or said it silently back then, because the punishment would have far outweighed any benefit. Still, internal cursing helped me get through many of life's trying moments in junior high and high school (if those boys who called me Donna Duck and Donnarhea could have heard the monologue in my head back then, they would have blushed).

But in all the times in my life that I have turned to cursing, I never found it to be such a gift as when I had cancer. Swearing was as much a part of my treatment protocol as chemotherapy was. You may find, too, that there are times when cursing is not only an *appropriate* response but quite possibly the *only* response.

Hey, I wouldn't be saying any of this if it weren't firmly backed in science: Researchers have studied cursing for decades, and they keep coming back with positive reasons to do it. Namely, swearing has been shown to relieve pain and improve our sense of well-being by elevating our endorphin production, which lowers our perception of pain. (If you're unfamiliar with endorphins, just know that they were named by smooshing "endogenous," meaning "produced within the body," with "morphine," meaning "see ya later, pain.") Swearing is an emotional release that leaves us calmer than we were prior to the swear. It also makes us feel more powerful, resilient, and in control.

I'm not suggesting that you break loose with a profanity-laced diatribe in the middle of a doctor's appointment, but some well-placed under-the-breath or right-out-loud cursing is a harmless way to blow off steam before the steam makes your head explode. (My personal favorite? "Fuck *me*." TRY IT. This particular phrase serves double duty: releases the pressure and then makes you chuckle — another endorphin-freeing action.)

My sister, not a big curser by nature, called to thank me for my swearing advice one day, because shortly after her mastectomy, swearing was the only thing that enabled her to get her bra and shirt on by herself. But don't take my word for it. In her own words: "I tried and tried, and almost gave up, but then I dropped an F bomb and suddenly found new strength. I hesitated at first, but then thought, 'Hey, Donna does it all the time. It works for her; maybe it'll work for me. And it *did!*'"

Debbie went on to explain that, in the face of frustration or fear, her go-to strategy had been singing a hymn she'd learned in church about being strong and pressing on. But on this particularly harrowing day, cursing seemed a more satisfying response. I say great on both counts! There comes a time in our lives when we find we need to use every tool in our toolbox. This is that time. Hymns, F bombs, chocolate, laughter — whatever gets you through the day is the perfect answer for *you*.

Things that go bump. Getting through the night can be a different story. While we're on the topic of fears, frustrations, and anxiety, let's talk about how things can change when the lights go out.

When you were a kid, nighttime could be scary, couldn't it? You'd try to put your active little mind to rest, close your eyes and start to wonder in the darkness: Is there a monster under the bed? in the closet? What was that sound? Is something — or someone — scary going to get me? For Deb and me, vampires and werewolves were always of primary concern. We watched "Dark Shadows" every afternoon after school and, as much as we loved the show in the light of day, its lingering memories could be horrifying at night. I tucked my sheets and blankets tightly under my neck so that, confronted with such an impenetrable barrier, head vampire Barnabas Collins would realize he had been outsmarted and move on to another, less prepared victim. (How I hoped it would not be Debbie, but hey, she knew the stakes when she opted to kick her blankets off in the middle of the night.)

Unfortunately, cancer might take you back to that scary nighttime place. By day, you may have no problem maintaining your positive mindset. But in the still of the night, the dark side of the disease — actually, the dark side of our psyches — comes to light. Monsters start popping out of the closet. Every doubt, fear, ache, and pain comes to the surface. Even if your prognosis is outstanding, the looming threat of your mortality can hang in the darkness like thick fog:

> *What's that twinge? Ugh. That's new. Am I hot?*
> *Damned docs have me paranoid about getting a fever.*
> *What did they say — go to the ER if it hits 100.4*
> *degrees? Or was it 104 degrees? How will I get to the ER?*
> *I won't be able to drive. Who will I call? Who can I call at*
> *3 in the morning? Am I going to die from this disease?*
> *What if I do — what will the kids do? How will they ever*

... oh, man, tomorrow morning I'm going to get all of my papers in order and make sure I put them in a visible place in case I die. Wait. I'm not going to die. Think positive, positive, positive. Visualize health. Visualize joy. Think happy thoughts. Who am I kidding? How can I think positive when I have a fever? Do I HAVE a fever? Where's my thermometer anyway?

Maybe it's just me, but it seems that at night, negative thoughts can swirl through our brains like a freaking tornado. It's not that we're not tired enough to sleep. We are most definitely tired. And we recognize that sleep is a gift to be treasured right now. If only we could turn off the negative thoughts. If only.

We can, of course. We are the ones allowing that doubting voice to enter our minds, so we can certainly stop it. It starts with recognizing what's going on and telling that voice inside your head to SHUT UP. I know. It's not as easy as it sounds, and if you're like me, it doesn't always work. I would push myself toward prayer and positive self-talk, but sometimes I'd positive talk myself right through to morning. Sleep would have been much nicer. Just keep trying, though. I promise you, things almost always look better in the morning.

For me, most of these unsettling nights happened during the months I was going through chemo. My guess is that a good part of the issue might have been the foreign substances floating around in there, but I also wonder if this dark-side soul searching might be just a normal part of the healing process. Maybe it's something we need to go through, playing out our scenario to its worst possible conclusion, whatever that happens to be in our respective minds, and then backing up from that to the relief that life really isn't that bad. Maybe this is what keeps pushing us back to our spiritual center of strength and motivates us to keep pressing on.

I honestly don't know. What I *do* know is that this phenomenon seems to be as much a part of the human condition as hope and faith are. Because we let darker thoughts enter our minds doesn't mean we don't believe. It just reinforces once again that we're human. We have weak moments. Fearful moments. Tearful, uncertain, self-pitying moments. And whether these come at night or at some other time, they may be as necessary to the healing process as our treatments, positivity, and prayer.

Dr. Lois reminded me many times that we need to give ourselves a break. She once told me quite scientifically, and I quote, "You're going through some heavy shit right now."

Amen, sister. Amen.

SURGERY, CHEMO & RADIATION

Chapter 7
The Boob Controversy

To re-breast or not to re-breast? There's a question I never expected to have to ask.

America is obsessed with breasts. You know, I've written this paragraph 15 different ways, only to find that these five words say it all. In fact, I can cut it down to three: America. Obsessed. Breasts. You know what I'm talking about. I mean, I recently saw an article about skin-tightening masks for breasts. Yeah. A little obsessive.

As I looked toward my mastectomy date, I conferred with several friends to see whether they thought it was necessary for me to get implants. Wouldn't it be healthier and more natural for me to just move forward and adjust to my new physique? I never quite understood the need to have amputated breasts replaced. I mean, if you have an arm removed, you lose a lot of functionality. A leg? Mobility. But boobs? Meh. They don't really hold much purpose beyond breastfeeding.

Don't tell men that.

"Wait, wh-… what are you asking me? You mean like you're considering not having anything there? No boobs? No boobs at all? No. That isn't right. You gotta have boobs," said every straight man I asked, apparently from some internal script that gets installed free with every heterosexual penis. In several cases, the color drained from their faces as they contemplated any outcome other than full breast replacement. One of my friends actually started pacing in circles. I fetched him a glass of water and apologized for my insensitivity.

I'd like to say women were more understanding, but, although they couched it in different terms, I got the same answer. "But isn't this an opportunity to get a free boob job?" they'd say, presumably to make me feel better. "I mean, if I had the chance to get bigger, perkier boobs, man, would I ever — especially if it meant getting rid of some of this fat from my belly or ass!"

Each time I smiled but wondered to myself *Would you really? Because I would really prefer to NOT be making this decision right now. Suddenly, my breasts seem to be the most beautiful breasts in the world exactly as they are!*

But we do have to make the choice as to if/how we will replace our breasts, at least when mastectomy is the plan. Most of us opt for reconstruction, if only because we want to feel as much like our precancerous selves as possible. For some reason, we believe that if we look the same, we will *be* the same. (Spoiler: You will *not* be the same after this experience. You will be better, stronger, and yes, more beautiful. More on that later.) We also don't want people to be uncomfortable looking at our concave chests. But do we really want to strap on a prosthetic every time we leave the house? Of course not. And so, many of us choose to re-breast.

Re-breasters have two choices:

1) We can have expanders put into place during surgery and then get biweekly saline fill-ups to stretch the skin gradually to the appropriate size for holding implants. (Expanders feel kind of like if you strapped mini backpacks to

your chest and filled them to bursting once every two weeks.) The swap-out with "permanent" (in quotes because they're not; they generally need to be replaced after a decade or so), usually silicone, implants happens later, once chemo and radiation treatments are done if you're having them.

2) We can have fat sucked from another part of our body and lopped into the new breast pits during the initial surgery. This option extends surgery and recuperation time, but it's a more natural and permanent solution.

This is why I say that others' comments are often underinformed. Women who think they would "give anything" for this "opportunity" don't realize what "anything" actually entails. We go through a lot of stuff people don't see unless they've had breast cancer themselves or accompanied a loved one who has. I'm sure that their intentions are good when they tell us that we should go to a tattoo parlor and have nipples inked onto our incisions to make our breasts look "natural," but I wonder how fast they'd be making that trip themselves.

As for me, I gave in to my focus groups and went with silicone implants — not the kind of porno-sized implants I'm sure some of my friends expected ("If I were you, I'd go big" — thanks for your input, Kevin), but smallish ones that resembled the real ones. I will admit: They made me feel better about my loss, because it didn't feel so much like there had been a loss.

As luck would have it, though, an incision failure set off a series of events that caused me to have to give up one of the implants. And while I could have elected to have both of them removed so I could at least maintain symmetry, temporary emotional instability prevented me from making that sound decision, and so the ordeal left me a little out of balance – yet still FINE.

The lesson is this: It all works out. Whatever your situation is, and whatever your choices are, just make the best decision you can and go with it. Some women get implants (with or without nipple tattoos) and live happily ever after. Others go breastless and are just as happy — maybe happier. I haven't met anyone else with one implant and one pit like me, but I'm sure others are making it work, too. Also: Have you seen the trendy full-chest tattoos that celebrate life after mastectomy? They can be gorgeous. Honestly, making this decision is like deciding to remodel your house. It'll never look quite like it used to, but you can still rock your own beautiful style.

Sorry: All this talk about bilateral mastectomy, and I've neglected the single mastectomy and lumpectomy crowds. Know that you're in good company in having your breast(s) altered, too. Here's where having friends who have been there is extremely comforting. One of my friends says that one of her nipples points up and the other down. Another reports that one of her breasts is now quite misshapen due to the removal of a tumor. And guess what? They are both completely happy with these inconsistencies, because they see the bigger picture.

Physical imperfections are a small price to pay for more healthy, happy days on this earth.

Chapter 8
Hospital Hijinks

Think of surgery as a much-needed nap. You'll have plenty of time to deal with the rest later.

If you've spent your life feeling fearful or nervous about hospitals, it's time to get over that. Easier said than done, I suppose. You walk in and sometimes don't know *what* is about to happen to you; how can you NOT be nervous? But here's what I can tell you: I've been sliced, diced, poked, prodded, punctured, injected and yes, even infected, but none of it was really that bad. It comes down to this: The people in the hospital — doctors, nurses, aides, whoever — want to help, not hurt, you. (Most of them anyway. My tale of Nurse Wretched, coming right up, is the exception rather than the rule.) So while you may fear the unknown, you need to have faith that fellow humans are there to hold your hand. If you're fortunate enough to have family or a close friend beside you as well, even better.

All you need to do to conquer your uneasiness is to get into the right mindset. Trust that whatever you're there for — tests, surgery, treatment — will put you one step closer to healing. Always go in with a positive attitude and see where the experience takes you. I promise you this: If things get a little rough, you will be amazed at how much strength you actually have inside. Plus, you'll have great stories to tell later.

If you're having surgery to remove a tumor or a breast or two, that's likely to be your most noteworthy hospital trip. If you get to stay a couple of days, you're in for quite a treat! Comic experiences, I'm talking, not an actual treat like an ice cream cone or something. But I know you'll have some fun with it.

I keep using words like "fun" and "funny," but you're probably thinking, *Um, excuse me, lunatic survivor, but I really don't believe that surgery is an innately "fun" experience.* And of course you're right. It's not. But with the right perspective, it's really not that bad. It's true that if you think about it too long, it'll freak you out. There's an easy solution for that: **Don't think about it too long!** My take is that the pressure isn't on you. It's on your surgical team. They do the work while you get to sleep. Who can argue with taking a good long nap? You'll have plenty of time to deal with the rest later. Remember, cancer is a one-step-at-a-time situation. First step of surgery? Take a nap. Woohoo!

As I've mentioned, I had a few cancer-related surgeries: the initial bilateral mastectomy and lymph node dissection, the swap-out of expanders for silicone implants, the replacement of the left implant when the incision split, and the subsequent removal of that implant when it became infected. So four, I guess. (My sister has had five, and I really hope she is writing her own book about … patience!) I'm going to tell you about the first one, because you can probably relate this more closely to your primary surgery.

What princess is wearing *this?* When I made trips to the hospital, I let curiosity drive my attitude. Hm, I wondered as I checked in for my mastectomy, will they let me see my room before I go to the operating room, like in a hotel? I could get myself settled in, stock up on ice, and maybe grab a bag of peanuts from the vending machine as I leisurely prepare for my big moment in the OR.

You might fantasize about vending machine snacks, too, because your surgeon will cut your food supply off the day before your surgery. If you haven't heard the term "NPO" yet, trust me when I tell you that you'll learn to hate it. We've all gone days when we don't necessarily eat a lot, but when someone tells you you're not allowed to eat, well, then it's all you want to do.

"What does 'NPO' mean?" I naively asked my plastic surgeon.

She smiled. "No soup for you!"

Well aren't you just a funny girl? I guess it's easy to crack wise quoting '90s sitcoms with a full belly. (If you're curious, NPO actually stands for *nil per os*, a Latin phrase that means, yeah, they're going to starve you until you emerge from the recovery room.)

So no peanuts or icy beverages — at least not yet. For now, it looks like I'm expected to take my clothes off in this cold, closet type of room. Then I have to remember what the nursing student said about how to put the gowns on. I can do that. Or can I? Wait. Does the blue floral gown go on first or second, forward or backward? And then, I don't know *what* I'm doing with the second one. What should I do with all of the random ties hanging from these not-at-all appropriately named "gowns"? I mean, what princess is wearing *this*? Also? What's with these slipper socks? They do have the hospital logo, which is kind of a nice touch. I had hoped for a souvenir.

All right. This is good: standing here shivering in my hospital-issued gowns that are layered front to back and back to front so that they choke me just a little, and white, chalky legs freezing as they spill into the logoed, cortical-grey socks. Apparently, I hadn't felt vulnerable enough, walking into the hospital to have my boobs cut off. I needed this. But come on, Donna: Think positive. Yes! I get it now. This is how they get you into the mindset of saying, "Do it! Just do it! Knock me out and wake me when it's over!" Hah! Clever of them, no?

Cool as a cucumber. When I checked back in with the nurse, she commented that she seldom saw people as relaxed and eager as I seemed to be for my surgery. I was just doing what I do — making jokes about the situation and answering her myriad questions as best as my middle-aged memory could. What year had my gallbladder been removed? *(Ummm….)* Was there any history of cancer in my family? *(Grab a scroll, my friend.)* How were my bowels functioning? *(PERsonal….)* Did I have any inkling were Waldo might be? *(I'm sorry, WHO now?)* These may not have been the exact questions, but you get the general idea.

Once I took my place on my assigned gurney, the witty writer checked in somewhere in the shallows of my mind and quipped, "Who named this bed on wheels? 'Gurney' has to be one of the butt-ugliest words ever created." She was right: I didn't feel special lying on that gurney slab at all, yet it seemed to me that I *should* feel special; I mean, cancer is kind of a big deal, right?

Next I remember a boy of maybe 14 years old sitting on a chair next to my gurney slab and assuring me he was with the anesthesiology team. I asked for I.D., not so much to see his affiliation with the hospital as to be certain he had cleared the seventh grade. He would be putting the IV needle into the back of my hand, he said.

"Awesome," I said. Next thing I knew, blood was pouring onto the floor. "Perfect," he said. "Really?" I said. "The blood is a very good thing," he said. "Are you a vampire?" I said. Visions of Barnabas Collins danced in my head as I felt consciousness leaving my body.

Love, love, love. As I understand it, my kids came to visit me in recovery, but I have no recollection of that whatsoever (drug-induced amnesia, I guess). Once they saw that I had lived through the hours-long procedure, they took their tired butts home to bed, leaving me in the loving care of my sister and brother-in-law.

I do remember seeing them, hustling down the hallway beside my gurney as the orderly whooshed me from the OR to my room. I recall chattering incessantly about who-knows-what, as some magical drug had me in a euphoric state. They stayed with me until I was situated and out cold once again. When I woke up this time, I saw they'd been replaced by my mom and dad, who were poised on the end of their visitors' chairs like children waiting for their turn on Santa's lap. I don't know how long they'd been sitting there at the side of my bed, watching me sleep, but their presence was a soothing comfort as I woke up in some state of confusion.

We chatted for a bit and then a nurse came bustling in with some beautiful flowers from one of my best friends. They brought happy tears to my eyes and, in that moment, I knew I was going to be all right. I might not have boobs anymore, but I sure had love.

Who's the nurse here? When Mom and Dad left, I examined my surroundings: hospital noises in the hallway, nurses scurrying back and forth past my doorway, and, of course, my beautiful flowers. I hurt a little. And it didn't take long before a nurse read me my rights about painkillers.

According to Nurse Wretched, "hospital rules" demand that the patient must request each and every dose of painkillers to get them. No matter how many times I think this through, I can't make the concept work in my head. Here's why: In the past, doctors have advised me to "stay ahead of the pain," by taking acetaminophen or another pain reliever on a regular schedule. "If you wait for the pain to intensify, it will be difficult to manage," they've always said.

But there I was, coming out of surgery and back to consciousness, and suddenly it was my responsibility to tell the nurse when it was time for my next dose. In essence, they're letting a person who is medicated to the point of drunkenness decide when it's time to "stay ahead of the pain." Mind you, the nurses will say no if your four hours haven't yet passed, which tells me that they KNOW when four hours has passed, so why don't they just give you the drug? Do they think you're scamming them to get the good stuff? That breast amputation is not a painful enough endeavor to merit some meds? All I wanted was to rest, without worrying about anything other than healing. Instead, I had to become a clock-watcher.

I try to give people the benefit of the doubt, though. Even in my slightly drunken and uncomfortable state, it was clear to me that the nurses were spread too thin. At one point, one of them came in and adjusted the IV tube in my hand. I realized moments later that it was now at an angle that had my IV solution dripping down my hand instead of going into me. I located the nurse call button and rang.

"Can I help you?" someone asked via intercom.

"My IV is leaking, and my bed is getting wet."

"OK. I'll have a nurse stop in."

Twenty minutes passed. Trust me on this: I had become adept at clock-watching (see above). I buzzed once again.

"Can I help you?" the voice said again, as if I had never contacted her the first time.

"My IV is leaking and my bed is getting wet."

"OK. I'll have a nurse stop in."

Third time's a charm, I thought, buzzing after another 15 minutes. This time, the nurse — *yeah, that one* — came in. She touched my sheet and said with disgust, "Did you wet the bed?"

Are you shitting me? I thought. Instead, I calmly replied, "No. When you adjusted my IV, it started leaking. I've been calling for help."

She became even more irritated by this. "Well, now how am I supposed to know how much of your antibiotic got into you? Why didn't you tell us sooner?"

The vacuum controversy. The day after my mastectomy, Nurse W. came in and asked if I wanted to go home. That was an option? It didn't seem like a good idea to me. I looked at my IV bag and wondered if I could take it with me. I stared at her blankly.

"Well, my mom had a mastectomy and went home and vacuumed the entire house that same day," she told me. Tears filled my eyes. *That is NOT true, you evil girl,* I wanted to say. *Your mom did no such thing, and how dare you imply that I'm a big, fat baby. Now wipe my tears.*

Maybe because she figured one less patient meant she might get a break today, this young nurse had adroitly planted the seed of doubt. *Was* I a big, fat baby? *Should* I go home? Had I overstayed my welcome already? "I…I guess I could go home," I said weakly. She smirked and walked away.

Shortly after, my surgeon — as mentioned before, one of kindest people I've ever met — showed up, interns in tow to gape at what was under the mummy-style bandage that encircled my now breast-free zone. After covering me back up, he asked, "What's this I hear that you're asking to go home already? You need to stay here and let us take care of you for a while. We can help you get stronger, and then you can go home. OK?"

I wanted to blurt out that I did NOT want to go home, that it was Nurse Wretched's idea for me to leave, and that she said I was a big, fat baby for not being at home cleaning my house. But I was too weak to reply. I simply nodded and tried to smile back at him.

Incidentally, when I was released from the hospital a few days later, the doctor specifically instructed, "Don't do anything strenuous for a while. No vacuuming or heavy lifting — nothing over three pounds."

Hey, where's that nurse? Did you hear that, girlfriend? No vacuuming. Boom.

Of course she was nowhere to be found.

Chapter 9
C Is for Chemo

The most unnecessary piece of advice I've ever received? No French kissing for 48 hours after chemo.

We've all heard the nickname "The Big C." Of course, it's not an endearing moniker; rather, one of those "If you don't say it aloud, then maybe it won't find you" kind of deals. And I get it — cancer has certainly earned that level of awe and respect — yet it's a different C word that commands my lifelong reverence: Chemotherapy (yes, with a capital C; if I could make it larger, I would).

Chemo is, in a word, badass. At once our best friend and worst enemy, it often brings us to our knees (sometimes literally, on those hug-the-porcelain days) before gently setting us upright again to continue on life's journey. Chemo is merciless in its attacks on cancer cells and, unfortunately, doesn't contain that ferocity as precisely as we might like. In other words, our healthy cells generally take a pretty good beating as well.

I'm not trying to scare you. In fact, I'm relatively sure that my bad time with chemo was an exceptional experience. My oncologist told me that it was unusual to see it hit someone so hard. That might have been her kind way of calling me a wuss, but that's OK. Today I feel fortunate that I experienced such a broad array of side effects, because I can help you prepare for whichever of the symptoms might affect you.

I started out with a very positive attitude on my first day in the "big chair." I met and instantly loved my chemo nurse, Stephanie, who became my advocate and friend throughout the duration of my treatments, which ended up lasting almost six months. Necessarily, Stephanie was a straight shooter. "You understand that this is poison, don't you, and that it will kill good cells along with bad?" she queried.

"I do, but let's not dwell on that and instead stick with the positive," I volleyed back enthusiastically. "That bag is filled with the magical elixir that is going to heal me. Bring it on!"

"OK," she said. "Here we go." (Was that blood I saw trickling from the tongue she was biting so hard?)

When I arrived for my second treatment, we exchanged a knowing look as I settled quietly onto the Throne of Torture. "One poison cocktail, please," I said, weakly raising my pointer finger.

I had not stopped believing in the healing powers of chemo — not for a single minute. I had simply replaced my naïve optimism with what I felt was a more realistic attitude. I knew in my heart that the treatments would heal me, but I also recognized that if I was going to come out of this experience whole, I needed to stand strong against the collateral damage. This was as close as I ever came to understanding the "fight" attitude so many people adopt with cancer. I mean, you give these chemicals the opportunity to share your body space, and they show their appreciation by gut-punching you. The phrase "Oh no you didn't" comes to mind.

If you've already started chemotherapy, then you might know what I'm talking about. If you haven't, don't be intimidated. I'll say once again that every person is different, and chemo affects every person differently. Also: Every *type* of chemo is different. There are many formulas and strengths, and what nauseates one person might not affect another at all. So, as you read ahead through some of my experiences, know that yours could be quite different. Quite better, I hope. Whatever your unique experience ends up being, just remember: You can absolutely do this. If I, wuss of wusses, made it through, you can, too!

Here's the thing: There's a laundry list of side effects that can come with chemo. I'm going to cover those I experienced myself. If you share in any of these experiences, then I hope you'll be comforted in knowing that you're not alone and that all of these can be overcome. If you *don't* experience some of these side effects, give yourself permission to gloat. *Hah!* you'll say. At least I don't have *that*. No one will hold this against you; you are welcome to any and every small victory you can claim along the way.

Before you go on: If you believe in the phrase "Pray for the best, but prepare for the worst," then go ahead and peruse this list. If you'd prefer to go into treatment completely unbiased, then skip over these to the next chapter, but know that they will be here if you want to compare notes later.

Alopecia. I'm starting with alopecia and giving it the most extensive coverage because it affects most of us who get chemo for breast cancer, and because we tend to be horrified at the thought of losing our hair. Baldness is for many of us a very significant are-you-shitting-me moment. *Let me get this straight,* we all say: *It's not enough that I have this [fill in your favorite expletive] disease; I have to lose my hair, too?*

Not if you believe the doctors. They'll tell you that not every woman loses her hair in chemotherapy. They're lying. Well, that's not fair. Let's say that they are supportively optimistic. But I have yet to meet a breast cancer patient who has made it through chemotherapy without losing at least a handful or two. Fact is, most of us lose it all — not only from our heads but from everywhere hair has ever lived on our bodies. For example, did you know that the tiny little hairs in your nose stop snot from pouring out of your head? They do. So when chemo takes those tiny little hairs, you can have quite the mess on your hands if you leave the house without a tissue tucked into your sleeve (I'm confident that this is nothing more than karma for making fun of our grandmas when we were young).

I know. It sounds gruesome. You like your eyelashes. And eyebrows. And headbrow. But don't panic. For one thing, they'll all come back. Once the chemicals are turned off, your body will start functioning as it did before. For another thing, by the time you're halfway through chemo, your hair will be the *last* thing on your mind. At that point, if someone questions your lack of luscious tresses, you'll just shake that shiny bowling ball and laugh.

The reality is that if alopecia is the worst side effect you experience, then you are truly blessed. Losing your hair doesn't hurt. It doesn't make you tired or nauseated. And it only makes you sad if you let it. Don't let it. Remember this: When your hair falls out, it's a victory. It means that the chemo is in your body kicking some serious ass. Embrace the experience, and take alopecia in stride. You have more important things to expend your energy on. Plus, you can grow new hair tomorrow. (Another glass half full? You can skip shaving your legs for a few months. Woohoo!)

In the meantime, you can address your baldness in a variety of ways. You can get a prescription for a "cranial prosthesis" from your oncologist (that's a wig, by the way, but the pretentious name apparently encourages insurance companies to bear a portion of the cost), you can wear hats, you can wear scarves, or you can be capital B-A-D and go boldly bald. I hold endless admiration for women with this level of confidence. I wish I had had the courage, but alas, I did not.

Instead, I went the scarf route. I tried cranial prosthetistry, but it always felt like I was peering out from behind some kind of annoying foliage. And then, maybe in some Freudian act of rebellion, I fried it in the oven. For real. No one tells you that you shouldn't bake while you're wearing the wig. Um, you shouldn't. I still picture myself cocking my head to one side in bewilderment as I tried to determine the source of the sizzling sound. That batch of brownies cost me $400.

Ten-dollar scarves started looking really good. They became my favorite solution to Med Head. They're easy and comfortable. Buy a handful of them in different colors and patterns, spend five minutes watching online videos on tying techniques, and you're set. I know what you're thinking: Scarves make some people uncomfortable because they wonder just what's going on with you. Does she have cancer? Is it her religion? Is she making a fashion statement? Eww, doesn't she wash her hair? Let 'em wonder. After one or two outings, you won't give it another thought, I promise.

Be patient with yourself, too. The first few weeks, I couldn't seem to tie a scarf onto my head without getting Shar Pei Forehead. Once I loosened up a little (yeah, literally loosened the tug while tying), I found that, for me, simpler was better. In fact, a few women at the cancer center even asked me to show them how to tie. It was the first time in my life anyone had asked me for fashion advice. Had I finally found my look?

Not if you ask my friend Edna. She came by shortly after I had shaved the few stragglers left on my head to take me scarf shopping. It was the first day I ventured out of the house with a scarf on my head, and I was feeling very self-conscious. I had bought only one to date — black, because I felt I needed to ease quietly into this new fashion statement. Edna took one look at me and said, "Good God, Donna, we need to get you something colorful. That black rag isn't doing you any favors. You look like death."

Although I thought she might have chosen her words a bit more carefully, deep down I knew Edna was right. The black *did* match the bags under my eyes and my chemo-grey skin, but it simply wasn't allowing my inner cancer glow to shine through. I started wearing more colors and patterns, and started feeling better about my appearance — most of the time. Not the time the little boy in the grocery store asked his mom if I was a pirate. That time, I was a little sad. But I shrugged it off, realizing that perhaps the large hoop earrings had been a bit of an overstretch given the whole scarf motif.

I'll leave this topic with an alopecia anecdote. Adam, who wanted to shave his head in solidarity with me (I convinced him otherwise, because I didn't want him to have to think about my disease every time he looked into a mirror), was talking with a friend whose mom had had cancer. She explained how her father had shaved his head in support. At a high school football game, the couple was in the stands, bundled for the chilly fall weather — she in a hat, he without. An acquaintance who hadn't seen them in a while came up to the man and shook his hand, saying, "Damn, Scott, look at you. Shaved your head, huh? You look great, man. I've thought about doing that myself, but I was afraid I'd look like a cancer patient." (Ba-dum-*CHING.*)

A final note: When your hair starts growing back in, you will be on top of the world. The first day I ventured out without my "cancer hat," I knew that I was doing it too soon. My aspiring flattop did not look even close to good. But suddenly I felt free, empowered in the knowledge that I had made it through the toughest part of the treatment, and I wanted to shout it to the world. Of course, to people who didn't know me, I was just a regular person who had made an unfortunate hair style choice. I could most definitely live with that. In fact, the idea made me giddy.

Well, as long as I started with the A word, alopecia, I might as well list the other side effects in alphabetical order. I'll be a lot shorter describing them, too, because I know you don't need a book on every topic!

Blurred vision. Although your vision might turn blurry and grow more so as your treatments progress, it should snap right back a few (three? six?) months after you're done. Be patient with your body and know that it's going to be OK.

Chemo brain. If you occasionally get mixed up, forget something that you really should have remembered, or just in general feel a little loopy during treatment, relax. People have been talking about chemo brain for as long as chemo has been the rage. Like blurry vision, it's temporary. As my great-grandma would say, *This too shall pass.*

Granted, if you have a "thinking" kind of job, chemo brain sucks in a big way. As a writer, I always made sure another writer or proofreader reviewed my assignments before they went out. Then, when I was deep into my treatments, I didn't do much creative writing work. And when I got to the final month or so of treatment and my confusion became pronounced, I didn't work at all.

"Adam, what day is it?" I remember asking at that time. "Tuesday," he said. Within minutes, I knew he had told me but I forgot, and that scared me. So I asked him again. "What day is it?" He repeated the answer, and this time I really focused on listening to him. Shortly after, panic set in as I realized I had forgotten yet again. On Take 3, he said, "Mom, are you playing with me?" As I looked into his face, I saw what I imagine I will see 30 years from now, when age gets the better of me. But not now, God, I thought. Please not today. Help me remember what day it is. Please. Help me come back.

Good news: I came back. Better news: You will, too. (Also? Chemo brain can be a gift. I don't remember throwing up after chemo at all. Rachel assures me, though, that she held my scarf back more than once. Bet *she* wishes for a bit of a memory lapse!)

Compromised immunity and anemia. While you're in treatment, you'll learn more about red and white blood cells than you've ever wanted to know. Unless you're in the medical field yourself, you might have to think back to biology class to recall that white blood cells stave off disease and red blood cells transport oxygen through your body. Chemotherapy hits both pretty hard. That's why your blood is tested before every treatment — to make sure your body is strong enough to get another dose.

If your white count drops, your immunity to diseases and infections may be compromised. During these times, you may need to wear a mask and gloves in certain environments. Don't hesitate or be embarrassed. Protecting yourself from germs is critical to your health and well-being. If it's your red cells that suffer, you might become anemic. For me, that just meant some shortness of breath and amplified fatigue, but sometimes it requires blood transfusions.

Again, I'm no doctor, so count on your chemo nurse and oncologist for information and guidance when it comes to your blood. They'll monitor it and help you understand the ups and downs.

Dehydration. Our entire lives, we've been told to drink eight glasses of water a day, and we say *Yeah, yeah. OK.* But then we don't do it. DO IT NOW. I'm not playing. During chemotherapy, water is precious because dehydration is dangerous. It can make you dizzy, weak, fuzzy-headed, and constipated like you never dreamed possible. Dehydration sends almost every chemo patient to the ER at one time or another. Something about the treatment sucks your body dry. Drink, and then drink some more.

My worst experience with dehydration happened one Saturday morning. I woke up and thought this must be what dying feels like. I had no idea how I was going to roll over, let alone get out of bed. My kids took me to the ER, where I was hooked up to one bag of fluids, then another. Within two hours, I was like new. In that moment, I realized how easy it would have been to avoid this situation. Just drink. Water, juice, a sports drink — whatever you can stand to suck down. But do *not* allow yourself to dehydrate.

In fact, whether you're in treatment yet or not, go get yourself a glass of water before you read on. I'll wait.

Eating issues. In chemo class, I learned that the typical breast cancer patient comes out of treatment about five pounds heavier than she went in. What? I was skeptical, because I had always heard that chemo makes you lose weight. Then I discovered that there are typically two phases of chemo for breast cancer patients. In Phase 1, you don't want to eat at all. In Phase 2, you will eat anything short of your own children.

Your chemo protocol might go differently, but at my hospital, the standard protocol that's administered begins with a formula patients have affectionately (and with spot-on accuracy) dubbed "The Red Devil." This part of the program, Phase 1, is where the reputation of nausea and weight loss was earned.

If you've ever been pregnant and tried to walk past the butcher's counter in your grocery store, then you know the kind of nausea I'm talking about. The thought of eating made my head spin. Salt and sugar might as well have been battery acid, and if anything had a smell, it wasn't getting near me. Remembering advice my mom had gotten from a friend who had for more than a decade taken treatments for bone cancer, I turned to mashed potatoes. "Eat something every day, no matter how bad you feel," Mr. Rigley had said, "even if it's just two bites of mashed potatoes." Mashed potatoes it was! I made a batch at the beginning of each week and ate a few bites with unsalted green beans or beets every day. (I'm not advocating for light eating at this time. If you can eat, EAT! My point is that you should never go a day *without* food. You need fuel to build strength.)

Then came Phase 2, the eat-everything-in-sight phase. You're ravenous because you take a steroid the day before your treatment to prevent an allergic reaction to the chemicals. Suddenly, you're on the opposite end of the spectrum. You become an eating machine. And just as you watched your weight spiral downward in the previous weeks, now you watch it climb. This is generally considered a blessing because, as you put on weight, you tend to feel a bit stronger. Another advantage of this phase of treatment is that the steroid wears on the day after your treatment, often energizing you to clean your entire house, weed all of your flower beds, and train for that half-marathon you've been dreaming about. Take it easy, though. Overexerting yourself is a surefire way of ensuring you'll be flat on your ass the next day.

Fatigue. Speaking of flat on your ass, I hate to deliver this news, but (big surprise if you've been living in a cave) there is a strong possibility that chemotherapy will at times make you tired. OK, maybe more than tired. You might have a couple of, or a few, days in each cycle when you feel like a cartoon character under a steamroller. I used to refer to these days as my time in "The Hole." When I was in The Hole, I couldn't socialize or eat. Watching TV was rough, and even listening could feel like sensory overload. It was like having a hangover and the flu at the same time. I could get up only to go to the bathroom, and that trip around the corner of my room was, well, a major trip.

I hope you never get thrown into The Hole. If you *do*, remember this: You *will* come out again! The secret is to be patient while time passes. My coping mechanism was to get through five minutes at a time, telling myself that I could do anything for five minutes, and after that time was up, I'd go through five more minutes, and then five more. I knew that with every brief stretch I was five minutes closer to being myself again.

Doctors and nurses tell you to get up, walk, and exercise, and that's great advice; it's just not always practical. The reality is that there may be times when you simply cannot move. Give yourself permission to rest! To quote Dr. Lois, "It doesn't mean you're not strong. It doesn't mean you're not brave. It just means you're human." To be completely transparent, I will tell you that I generally spent three or four days of each two-week cycle in bed, and by the time I got into my final treatments, the cumulative effects of the chemo left me flat with fatigue most of the time.

It's not pleasant, but it is absolutely doable, and the reward is very shiny in the distance. Keep your eyes on the prize. Hang in there, get through the next five minutes, and know that every treatment you put behind you puts you one step closer to the finish line.

Incontinence (I'm SORRY!). Toward the end of my treatment, I started losing bladder control — not in a major way; there was no all-out pants peeing. But my muscles were weak, and when I had to go, speed was of utmost importance.

One of the chemo nurses assured me that incontinence was not on the list of side effects for this treatment. "Well, you better add it then," I said, making intense eye contact so she'd know I was sincere. She suggested I try doing some kegels because, after all, women my age sometimes tend to start losing bladder control. Yes, I'm sure it's my age and not the fact that toxic fluids have been coursing through my veins for the past five months. Let me just go home and start doing those 10-second squeezes. What do you think, Marjorie? 20? 30? How many do *you* do? How's *your* bladder control? (Man, prolonged physical weakness can make you mean!)

I asked Mary Jane if she had ever lost bladder control while she was on chemo. "Of course," she said. "But don't worry. It comes back once your chemo's done." I told her what the nurse had said about kegels. We laughed until we peed.

Menopause. No woman wants to go through menopause, especially not before her time. But if someone tells you that it'll help prevent a breast cancer recurrence, I'm betting you'll get on board the Hot Flash Express in a hot minute.

I did.

In many cases, including mine, estrogen fuels breast cancer. Progesterone can, too. Since these hormones are produced and released by ovaries, doctors strive to shut the ovaries down, through chemo, radiation, and sometimes even surgical removal. Success in stripping these organs of their cancer-feeding potential means that menopause isn't far behind.

So we get hot flashes. Which suck. And can go on for years. But in the scheme of things? They're not so bad when you think they could keep you cancer-free. Also remember that another year of hot flashes is another year alive. Not a bad trade-off. So invest in a little fan, flip the switch when the fire starts, and smile, knowing you're starving that beast that tried to destroy you.

Metal mouth/Cabbage tongue. "Your mouth will taste like metal" chemo veterans told me, so I prepared by purchasing the requisite plastic forks and spoons. This turned out to be a good investment in that I did occasionally taste metal. What did I taste *all* the time? Cabbage. I could brush, floss, and swish all I wanted. That cabbage aftertaste just kept coming back.

I thought back to one of the rules I learned during the mandatory chemo class I had attended prior to starting treatment: *no French kissing for 48 hours after treatment.* This was one of the most unnecessary pieces of advice I have ever received, because (a) oddly, the chemo experience didn't leave me feeling particularly romantic, and (b) men weren't falling over one another to get with the woman without eyebrows, hair, and boobs. Oh, and with cabbage breath. Go figure.

Nausea. I said most of what I have to say about nausea in the "eating issues" entry. What can I tell you that you haven't heard from a hundred chemo patients before? Nausea is extremely common. It can range from a little wooziness and loss of appetite to all-out heaving. I never really found the trick to quelling these attacks, but the five-minute exercise I outlined under "fatigue" helped a lot!

Neuropathy. Tingly or numb fingers and toes go with the territory. You might experience this neuropathy during treatment or months after. I felt it slightly while I was in treatment, but thought that, for the most part, I had escaped its prickly grip. Then one day, when chemo and radiation were nearly invisible in my rearview mirror, I got up from my desk to get a glass of water and fell flat on my face. I stayed there for a minute trying to appreciate what had just happened, then laughed hysterically and said right out loud to no one, "And there it is."

Since then, I've been careful about holding expensive wine glasses or vases. And I stub my toes a lot. You don't realize they're there, so you can kind of trip over yourself. Just take things a bit more slowly than you did before. This is a manageable and generally mild piece of collateral damage. I've come to think of it as something of a badge of honor for survivors. We're tingly, baby. Effervescent.

But, yeah, we do drop a lot of stuff, too.

Tinnitus. OK, I'm starting to feel guilty about the length of this list, so I'll keep this super short. You might experience ringing or pressure in your ears. Try moving your focus away from the ringing. Music and conversation can help. But, like neuropathy, tinnitus might stick with you for a while. Be patient and positive!

Weak, weird nails. Your finger- and toenails might turn dry, thin, brittle, and weak. They might look weird for a while, and they might stay this way. But unless you're a hand or foot model, this probably won't cause much in the way of distress for you. I get over it by using strengthening nail polish. Easy fix.

No matter what side effects you might experience before, during, or after chemo, just remember to keep your head in the right place, hold on to that faith, and remember that almost all of these are temporary. Five minutes from now, your world is likely to feel much better.

FlatTop

Chapter 10
Radiation: That Special Glow

With its bright blue, purple, and green markings, my chest looked like a kids' board game.

Radiation can come at different stages in the journey. Some people have it before surgery to shrink their tumors. Others have it after surgery or after the surgery-plus-chemo combo, as kind of a clean-up crew to fry the cancer cells that were too stubborn to be pried off with the knife or washed away by the chemicals. Still others don't need radiation at all.

If radiation *is* part of your treatment protocol, never fear: It might be the easiest part. From my perspective, as well as that of many women I've talked with about it, it offered a relatively restful period following the intensity of surgery and chemo.

First, a comment on the entertainment value of the radiation experience: While I recognize that this is a very serious element of treatment, it is also possibly the most interesting part. If you go into this experience with the curiosity of a child, you won't be disappointed! Your body is colorfully marked, you're positioned somewhat like a pig on a spit under radiation-delivering equipment, and the machine itself looks like something from a spy movie, with clearly marked targeting tools that focus on your trouble areas like a sniper's sight. Yet you feel no pain or danger. If you go in with the right perspective, you can actually relax through your treatments.

In my treatment saga, the initial consult with the radiation oncologist was followed by an appointment to be "marked." This was a comfortable, noninvasive procedure during which a medical practitioner armed with permanent markers drew Xs, circles, and lines across my breasts (then expanders), chest, and sides to guide the radiation technicians to zap the right spots. For the most important Xs, she applied clear adhesive stickers to protect these marks from being washed off in the shower. These would remain in place throughout the six weeks of treatments.

When I got home, I took a look in the mirror and was taken aback by the surreal image. With its bright blue, purple, and green markings, my chest looked like a kids' board game or a complex trick play mapped out in a coach's playbook. I grinned at the silliness of it all but then felt a twinge of self-pity as I reminded myself that this wasn't a game. I wondered for a moment how I had gotten to this place. Then I remembered that this was the homestretch. I smiled again and went into my first treatment with renewed energy and resolve.

The instructions during treatment were simple enough: Lie still and hold on to the vertical steel pole above your head to expose the game board to the zapping device — a large overhead machine similar to an X-ray machine that my research tells me is called a linear accelerator, or LINAC. I realized that the requirement to hold this position for the 15 minutes or so of zapping was the reason my doctors had been so intent on an arm-exercise regimen after surgery. At every appointment, they'd ask me to raise my arms as high as possible. They weren't pleased that I hadn't been as good as I could have been about actually doing those exercises. Climb the wall with my hand? Absolutely not. My surgery left the nerves in my left arm raw, and certain movements gave me "zingers," so this arm exercise was low-grade mental and physical torture to me. But not doing it made my spit-stance on the radiation table a little tougher, so I do strongly encourage you to exercise your arms as much as possible in the weeks leading up to your time on that table.

The good news about radiation treatments is that this zapping doesn't hurt at all! In fact, if my armpits hadn't occasionally felt like they were on fire and my usually pasty-white skin hadn't turned charcoal black and peeled off in tiny sheets during the last week or so of treatments, I would've told you I wasn't even certain they had done anything to me. The uncomfortable effects to my skin really weren't bad or long-lasting. My radiation oncologist prescribed a soothing cream. Organic lotions helped, too.

As far as other side effects, I just got a little tired a few weeks into the treatments. The effects are cumulative, so that's to be expected. If you have chemo first, you may find that the tiredness from radiation is a far cry from the fatigue of chemo. (Before all of this, I had thought that tiredness and fatigue were one in the same. Not so. Tiredness is wanting a nap. Fatigue is being so exhausted that it's difficult to nap.)

I've never talked with anyone who had more intense side effects than tiredness and skin irritation, but I'm sure your radiation oncologist will give you the full rundown of possibilities. Hopefully, it will be an easy experience for you — one that contributes to your full recovery!

HEALING

Chapter 11
Physical Healing Starts Here

Be patient, loving, and kind to your body.

Even though surgery, chemo, and radiation are primarily in your doctors' hands, you play a starring role throughout your treatment protocol. That's because it's up to you to do not only the "hanging in there" but also the healing. The more active you are in this process — engaging body, mind, and spirit — the faster you will heal.

My comfort level in addressing healing is on the spiritual side. That's where I found my strength and why I've written several chapters about that aspect. But please understand that my intent is not to downplay the importance of the physical. It's a critical piece of healing. I just know that there are people far better qualified to advise you about this — members of your medical team, dietitians, personal trainers, and others who know the science behind what makes a body tick. Did I get through the physical aspects of healing? Yes. Was I an exemplary student of physical healing? No. So reach out to the experts for advice in regaining your physical form and function. Of course, you can count on me for a few personal notes.

WHAT the hell. When you come home from surgery, you will get a set of instructions including things like emptying your drains. Ummmm, let me see: Yeah, yeah, yep, this is as bad as it sounds. Worse really. You have plastic grenade-type receptacles hanging from your armpit(s) or side(s) that are attached to drainage tubes installed during surgery to pump excess fluids away from the surgery site. (I was at once fascinated and horrified that these run from inside your body to outside, right through your skin, like an electrical cord coming out of a vacuum.) It's your responsibility, several times a day, to empty the grenades (which you'll either have pinned to the inside of your shirt or stuffed into a pocket), measure their contents, and record those measures, along with the color of the drainage [pause for groan], on a chart.

I know. It's gross. However, it's probably the grossest thing you'll have to do through this whole process, so now at least you don't have to worry about being caught off guard. Also? This is a good chance to find out who your true friends are. For me, Rachel and Deb were stalwart soldiers in this special-duty assignment. They helped when I had trouble reaching, and almost never gagged — at least not in front of me.

OK, this might be more appealing. You'll also need to attend to incision care and bandaging, but that's easy stuff, plus you need to eat right (lots of protein, everyone told me), drink plenty of fluids, and exercise as much as you possibly can.

I mentioned in the previous chapter that one of the exercises your doc is likely to recommend is the "wall crawl," which requires you to essentially make your hand a spider and take it up the wall. And though this sounds innocent enough, if you've had a lymph node dissection, spider-crawling might bring on zingers, those nails-onchalkboard pierces of pain that send your brain straight to your cursing library (see Chapter 6 for ideas). Fortunately, zingers leave as quickly as they arrive. Unfortunately, they condition us to recoil from our arm exercises like the Frankenstein monster from a bonfire.

There are a whole series of arm exercises, though, and not all are as intimidating as the spider crawl. My advice is to be brave and do as much exercise as you can without placing undue stress on your psyche. Even as a cowardly exerciser, I ultimately regained full range of motion in both arms, but it took time. I'm betting you could get there faster with more exercise.

Chemo healing is its own thing. I talked a lot about chemo back in Chapter 9, so I'll keep this short. How can you honor your body during chemo so that you bounce back as soon as you can? DRINK. I know I emphasized this before, but if I said it on every page, it still wouldn't be enough. Dehydration happens fast and hits you like a train. Drink as much as you can, striving for a half-gallon a day. Also eat healthy foods and remember on those days you don't want to eat that even a little food each day will help sustain you.

Once again, it's important to exercise any time you feel strong enough. Engage in the physical activities you're comfortable with. Getting back to your exercise routine, even though you'll need to modify it, is important for your body and spirit. I found walks in the fresh air to be exhilarating and empowering, as long as I took along plenty of water. I'll caution you, though, that you need to stop when you get tired. I walked too far one hot summer day and ended up needing to call a friend for a ride home. Then I was flat in bed for a day. Find your balance and know your limits. You can't force yourself back to health.

Testing your patience. This brings me to my final point about physical healing — the whole "patience is a virtue" thing. Sometimes when you think you're done, you're not quite done. There could possibly be loose ends to tie up in the months that follow, because the nature of life is that things don't always go 100 percent according to plan.

You can approach these situations one of two ways: You can say, *NO, NO, NO! I'm done. Can't do any more. Won't do any more. Go away.* OR you can, once again, dig deep into your soul and persevere in the knowledge that you possess amazing strength of body and spirit, and that you will navigate this twist in the road with precision and expertise. Look at all you've done so far!

If your challenge is that your cancer is metastatic, then it's obviously much more than a "loose end," and you're probably already working on a plan to manage your disease. Having not been in that position myself, I wouldn't be so arrogant as to try to offer advice. I would, though, ask that you consider documenting your journey as you move forward so that you can not only take comfort in your victories along the way but also serve as a role model for the rest of us. Your strength and insight will become the inspiration and direction for those striving to navigate that same road, and they will channel that strength right back to you when you need it. We are light-years stronger when we stay connected!

If your challenge is smaller — an issue with your reconstruction, for example — then try to put it into perspective. When you really think about it, this challenge is probably not of the same caliber as what you've already been through, so just hang in there a little while longer, and keep your eyes on the prize.

Deb and I both had issues with our healing and reconstruction, which at first we thought was quite the coincidence. But as we've talked with more and more women, we've found that it's relatively common to need surgical "revisions." Sometimes the incision just doesn't hold, or other issues develop.

I mentioned earlier that I had challenges with my left side. Basically, my incision split after my implants were in place, so I had a new surgery, with a new implant, but the incision became infected — twice. The first time I spent three days in the hospital getting IV antibiotics to clear it up. Then, for several weeks, I would spend two hours a day in a hyperbaric oxygen chamber breathing pure oxygen as an additional healing measure. Unfortunately, when another tiny tear appeared in the incision, I had to have the implant removed for good. Apparently, the fat layer under my skin had been virtually eliminated due to the large amount of radiation administered to clear my chest wall of cancer cells, and now my skin is too thin to hold an implant. I get it. I had wanted the strongest treatment possible, after all. But this situation did call for a lot of patience.

Deb was even more patient than I was, as she experienced various thises and thats that led to a total of *five* surgeries. She could have given up at any time in the process, but she persevered and now looks back at her experience feeling victorious.

My point in sharing our stories isn't to scare you that something like this will happen to you. It probably won't. But if it does, don't get discouraged. If we can do it, you can do it! I considered my issues nothing more than hiccups along the way. Always come back to that bottom line: You are alive and, hopefully, on your way back to health. In the overall scheme of things, these are minor setbacks. The important thing to remember is that you should always be patient, loving, and kind to your body and spirit. They've been through a lot.

Chapter 12
Spiritual Healing 1: People and Their Gifts

Gifts are a spiritual bond that connects us.

Sometimes we get so caught up in the physical healing that we neglect working on the vital psychological, emotional, and spiritual healing. But I'll tell you this: On those days when I felt too tired to move, what got me back on my feet again were conversations with the people I love, crayon drawings on my wall from my great-nieces and nephews, joyous photos of my family and friends, and the selfless outpouring of support from virtually everyone I know through cards and gifts that reminded me we were all in this thing together.

To set the record straight, I've never been big on material things. If my home is warm and cozy, it doesn't matter if it's a mansion or a rented room in someone's upstairs. And my car's entire job is to get me there, not to impress anyone or break performance records. But there's a difference between material goods and the gifts people give you. As it turns out, gifts can impart great healing strength. That's because they hold the intentions of the people who are giving them. Here's what I mean:

My Aunt Helen, who was the embodiment of the phrase *joie de vivre*, crocheted an afghan for me when I was a teenager. I knew at the time that this was a special labor of love, but I didn't realize how important this blanket would come to be later in my life. I remember feeling very special when Aunt Helen gave me the choice of black or white granny squares, with any color flower I'd like. I chose black with bright yellow flowers, each trimmed with four small green leaves. I cherished this gift and, through the years, wrapped myself in it anytime I needed comfort, or when I missed my dear aunt, who passed away when I was in my early 20s.

Aunt Helen's afghan became a source of comfort as well as connection and healing for me, not only because of all the love she crocheted into it but also because both she and her sister, my Aunt Mary Kay (aka *Babe*), were important role models for me. Sadly, they had each walked their own cancer journeys at a time when medicine simply wasn't up to the task. They came to know the depths of this disease in a way I have not; remembering their courage helped me ratchet up my own. I held them both close in spirit as I navigated each day.

Then there was Edna, who made me a beautiful quilt in healing, soothing yellow and lavender (she is a genius with fabric). She took the additional step of taking it to her yoga/Reiki studio and asking everyone there to pray over it for my health. I kept this blanket, along with Aunt Helen's afghan and a wonderful purple prayer shawl from my friend Dan's church on my bed as constant reassurance that I wasn't in this alone. Running my hands over the soft quilted fabrics or snuggling under the layers of warmth sustained me in even my weakest moments.

I got some awesomely fun and funny gifts, too, in addition to a wide range of practical solutions to the issues I faced. My friend and business partner Tom, a very talented designer, created a T-shirt for me with my own logo — *WHTFTS?* (Who Has Time For This Shit?) — which I wore on days when I was feeling sassy (or riding the high of the chemo steroids), and my friend Doug gave me honeycomb from one of his own beehives, which was a symbol of promise for the future (anecdotally, honey has preventive/curative properties including some related to blocking cancer recurrence, so, yeah, bring it on!). One of my neighbors, Sue, who had gone through breast cancer herself, presented me with a fabulous "Box of Sunshine," a dozen or so fun and helpful items that were all bright yellow to add cheer to my days.

I was overwhelmed by the thought and spirit that went into these gifts and so many others, from beautiful hats, scarves, and a satin pillowcase that cradled my bald head, to button-down shirts that made dressing so much easier after surgery (my friend Robin actually went out shopping for me and sent a crateful of gorgeous clothes from halfway across the country), a comfortable lounge chair for soaking up the warm summer breeze (this gift from my brilliant friend Darlene became my "healing chair"), and homemade dinners that comforted my soul. (So. Many. Delicious. Dinners.) Every gift I received touched my heart.

I'm sure you're finding this, too — that the gifts people give you are filled with love and positive energy, whether they are something they made for you, something they thought you'd like because they know you so well, or something they like themselves that they hope will bring *you* the kind of comfort it would bring *them*. The intentions behind these gifts are precious. Keep them nearby. Touch them. Hold them. Reread every card and handwritten note. Feel the spiritual hug, and recognize that these material things are physical manifestations of the spiritual bond that connects us, holding us together as we feel the visceral tug of our collective humanity and stand united in our faith.

Gifts and cards are constant reminders that you are not overcoming this disease just for yourself; you're doing it for every friend, every family member, every neighbor, and every colleague who is rooting for you. For the most part, people give because they love and care about you. But there's also a tiny part that reflects the giver's awakened sense of their own mortality. Through you, they seek the reassurance that they will have the strength, too, if ever faced with a similar diagnosis. And so, through the transfer of gifts and prayers, *your* health becomes *their* well-being.

If you've always been the giver and never the receiver, it's time for you to open up to the idea of accepting gifts without hesitation. It's not just about comforting yourself, although that is a tremendous benefit of gifts. It's also about instilling joy and hope in those who give to you. Even as you might yourself be lying nauseated in bed, you are healing someone else by giving them the opportunity to feel helpful and needed. And when you regain your health, your victory will be theirs as well — fist bumps, high-fives, and celebration all around.

Chapter 13
Spiritual Healing 2: The Joy of Music

Charms to soothe the savage breast? You bet.

I come from a long line of dancers. Not professional dancers, mind you, but dancers who shake their booties for the sheer joy of it. Some of my happiest childhood memories are of my four aunts — Pearl, Ruth, Helen, and Babe — dancing "like no one was watching." I would look forward to our summer family reunions, hosted in my mom and dad's pavilion, because I knew those parties would be filled to the brim with high-energy music and dancing. The Wodianka sisters never disappointed, as they would clap their hands and shake it, A-line shirtdresses swishing tirelessly to the rhythm.

My parents were no slouches on that worn wooden dance floor, either. Their jams tended to be cha-chas and jitterbugs. My mom would delight in the spirit of the dance, while my 6-foot-3 giant of a dad surprised me every time, dancing with a level of grace that was completely out of character for the truck-driver persona we saw every other day of the year.

It was only natural that when I grew up to be a mom, I would comfort my babies by dancing with them. (No surprise either that Adam became a musician, although where the heavy metal came from remains a mystery.) Dancing became such a bright spot in my days that I've committed to it ever since. At my most recent checkup, my doctor asked me about exercise.

"Do you exercise every day?"

"Absolutely."

"What kind of exercise do you do?"

"Well, I walk."

"Great."

"I work with small weights."

"Good."

"And I dance."

"I'm sorry, what?"

"I dance."

"You *dance*. [Her scribe looked at my menopausal physique and snickered.] What kind of dance?"

"The kind where you move your arms and legs, wiggle your butt — you know, *dance*."

Pause for pin-drop.

"What? Is that weird?"

"No! No, it's great. It's just that most people don't *dance* every day."

"Well, maybe they should."

Mm, hm. They should. You should, I should, we all should dance — and sing. You know why? Because music heals.

Have you ever found music to be helpful during stressful times? I'm guessing so. You probably know that's because music triggers dopamine, the feel-good hormone that brings about a sense of bliss. When we listen to music we love, it helps us feel better about things and encourages us to relax and breathe. It also has the power to bolster your courage, energize you, or lull you to sleep, depending what kind of support you need at the moment. Think about it: How can negative thoughts overrun your mind and spirit when you're listening to your favorite music?

And so music is the ideal healing force for you to tap into right now. Don't limit yourself to passively listening; when you can, participate. Sing! Dance! Play that air guitar! The inherent joy of music knows no bounds. Nor should you. If you feel well enough to dance, cut loose! I sang and danced through cancer whenever I had enough energy, and it truly lifted me up. If you find yourself humming along with a classic, grab that hairbrush microphone and belt it out, baby! Fuel your soul with melodic energy, off key or on — makes no difference. Music is joy. Joy is healing.

Another great thing about music is its portability. You can take it with you to the hospital and chemo treatments as easily as you can listen to it at home. That gives music the potential to be your constant companion, always at your fingertips, poised to play whatever you want whenever you want. Let it soothe you, empower you, and surround you with light!

Here's an extra idea for tapping into the power of music: Choose a victory song — something upbeat and audacious. You might already have a song in mind, or it might come to you seemingly out of nowhere. (I heard "Rock Me Amadeus" at a couple of pivotal moments, and it stuck.) Keep your song close and use it to celebrate every victory along the way, no matter how big or small. This song will stay with you long beyond your cancer journey. It will buoy your spirit and fuel your faith every time you hear it, reminding you to celebrate *you* — your life, your health, and your happiness.

Chapter 14
Spiritual Healing 3: Should You Try Reiki?

Comfort, relaxation, peace — I'm sorry. What was the question?

A decade ago, medical practitioners didn't talk much about Reiki as part of a healing protocol. Energy work of any kind was pooh-poohed by most because it didn't fit within the guidelines of Western medicine. But stories started emerging of patients who were finding relief in Reiki. Research followed and confirmed that positive changes were happening. Now, health systems across the country are providing or suggesting Reiki treatments as a supplement to traditional medical protocols.

In my book, this is a very good thing.

If you're unfamiliar with Reiki [RAY-kee], it's a Japanese word that basically means "universal life energy," referring to the energy that flows through all living things.

A trained, certified Reiki practitioner won't profess to be a healer but rather a channel through which this energy freely flows. By touching or nearly touching you with their hands, Reiki practitioners infuse your body with positive energy. It's noninvasive and nonchemical, yet it holds the potential to be transformational.

Most people describe Reiki treatments as calming, relaxing, and comforting. In my experience, Reiki was much more than that. It was life-changing. My first treatment went something like this:

I had been through three cycles of chemo, and my white count was so low that it was questionable whether I'd be able to take my next infusion on time. Edna had told me about the amazing experiences she had had with Reiki treatments at a studio called Branches of Wellness, so I asked her to take me there. One of the Reiki masters greeted us warmly and took me into a small room that smelled of incense and hope.

I slid onto the table and lay silently in my clothes and headscarf, covered with a warm blanket, eyes closed under a soothing, weighted eye mask. The Reiki master proceeded to place her hands lightly on or over various spots on my body, spending several minutes on each area. I slipped without effort into a quiet, meditative state, feeling peace and comfort envelop me. I had no idea how much time had passed, but when she had finished, I was more relaxed than I could remember having been ever before. I opened my eyes and sat up to listen to her report of what *she* had experienced during the session. (Because they are sharing your personal energy space during the treatment, Reiki practitioners often pick up vibes about your health — they may sense where the flow of energy is blocked or slowed down in your body, for example, which enables them to channel additional energy to those areas. Some may also receive spiritual messages or visions that help them provide more insight.)

She shared that she had felt love and support all around us. She described my grandfather, explaining he had been standing at my head, praying over me and vowing to stay with me through whatever challenges lay ahead. There was a grandmotherly figure, too, she said, along with other relatives, healing souls, and angels. Tears sprang to my eyes as I was overcome by this outpouring of pure, unconditional love. In this moment, I knew that if I were to be physically healed of this disease, it would be through the blessings of these loving spirits, and that if I were not to be physically healed, then they would guide me with comfort and love into the next world. Either way, I was completely at peace.

I left the studio energized and elated. The next day at the cancer center, my white count was so high that they checked it twice to make sure the lab hadn't made a mistake. No mistake. My Reiki session had caused a dramatic and measurable physical improvement. If I had ever had a doubt about whether spirituality plays a role in health, it disappeared with that blood test. And while I understand that not every Reiki treatment will bring about such profound results, I say why not give it a try? Worst case, you relax and get some much-needed rest. Best case, you leave stronger than you ever dreamed possible.

YOUR NEW NORMAL

Chapter 15
Of Mountains and Molehills

A group of 80-somethings are enjoying brunch. "How have you been feeling, Dorothy?" one of them asks. "Like a million bucks," Dorothy answers. "Of course, if I had felt this way 30 years ago, I would have called an ambulance."

Friends and family would often ask, "How's the book going?" I would wince knowing I'd have to see their disappointed faces when I replied, "It's … going." I didn't know why I couldn't seem to wrap it up, but I just couldn't. Then I discovered why. I wasn't ready yet. I didn't understand something of critical importance to our story line.

You see, I had planned to write this chapter, this introduction to the new normal that comes after surgery and treatment, by explaining that a lot of compromises might be in order — that you might have to get used to the idea that your body may not always work the way you'd like it to, and that you might have to limit some of your activities and curb some of your dreams. Then I had an epiphany. On a mountain. A mountain I climbed. Suddenly I had a whole new perspective to share with you.

Now, when I say I *climbed* a mountain, understand that I am totally overdramatizing the situation. If you pictured me geared up with harnesses, ropes, and carabiners, shake that image right out of your head. I didn't dangle from ledges before I had cancer; I certainly wasn't about to dangle afterward. I don't even own real hiking boots. What I actually did was hike up a mountain trail in my tennis shoes. It's also only fair to tell you that this wasn't a big mountain. It was a small mesa in Colorado, where my son Adam lives. Nonetheless, it was a mammoth challenge to me, not only because of my recent bout with disease, but also because my Ohio lungs had in no way adjusted to the thin air.

Adam was a saint that day. He could have easily jogged to the top had I not been in tow. Instead, he coached and encouraged me to take it one small stretch at a time until we made it up and over the top. "See that little tree up ahead, Mom? That's as far as we need to go before you can rest." We'd get to the tree, and I'd be huffing and puffing while he'd say, "Look — you did it! Now just catch your breath. We're in no hurry." We'd get to another small tree, and then a big rock, and then some kind of unusual Colorado plant that I'd take some time examining, more out of necessity than curiosity. Step by step, yard by yard, five minutes by five minutes, we climbed that trail until we finally reached the top.

Twirling around so I could get the 360 view of the majestic landscape — snow-capped mountains, explosive white clouds, and skies as blue as I had ever seen — I wept. Pumping my fists into the air as high as I could lift them, I shouted, "Cancer? I hardly know her!"

This awe-inspiring moment etched a vital message into my soul as I stood on top of that beautiful mesa: No matter how broken we might become or perceive ourselves to be, we always have the capacity to emerge whole again. Our wounds simply allow more light and love in, giving us the opportunity to immerse ourselves more deeply in life than we ever have before.

Life is different physically. Yes, there are day-to-day challenges that are likely to be part of your new normal, because surgery, chemo, and radiation are tough on our bodies. But when our spirits are powered by our inner mountain climber, and when we treat ourselves with patience, love, and respect, we can handle any changes to function or form our bodies might sustain.

Docs will tell you to give your body a year to reboot. That's good advice. And if you've had chemo, remember that that stuff stays in your system for a long time, so you might think that a symptom is part of your new normal when it's actually just chemicals still working their way out. Don't panic if your memory really stinks for a while, or if your vision is blurry. If you have neuropathy, just be careful holding glasses and vintage vases, and be aware that you might trip over your feet now and then. You also might have random phantom itches that you can't relieve. And osteoporosis or osteopenia might make you feel a little creakier than when you started.

Also, if your doc prescribes an estrogen-blocking medication to reduce the risk of recurrence, give it a good six months before you judge whether or not it's right for you. I've heard that many women give up on it because of the side effects (namely bone pain), but I think if they knew that those symptoms would likely subside in a few months, they might stick with it. Remember once again that every drug is different with every body. Some women never have a single symptom on this type of drug. Others continue to have side effects after several years. My experience fell in between. For five months, every bone in my body ached, and I'd be up roaming the floors at 3 a.m. But I stayed with it, and by month six, the pain began to subside. I started sleeping through the night again, and today I feel no pain and I'm so happy that I didn't give up!

One more thing: Make sure that you get every medical checkup and follow-up test your doctors recommend, and stay in tune with your body so you know when something is amiss. On the other hand, don't allow yourself to become paranoid about a recurrence. Without exception, every survivor I've ever talked to on this subject says that their mind goes there sometimes when they get sick or suffer aches or pains. *Is my cancer coming back?* we wonder. But while this thought might be a new "reflex" for you, don't let it haunt you. Your body got sick before cancer; it will also get sick after cancer. That doesn't mean that the illness is *caused* by cancer. Still, if you have an ailment that sticks around for a while, have it checked out. (Always respect the power and potential of the C.)

Physical challenges hanging on? Put them into perspective. Embrace them. They are mementos of your courageous journey. Take a deep breath and ask yourself this: *Am I grateful to be alive? To be able to create more moments, more memories? To smell coffee in the morning and flowers in the spring?* Your new normal is your reminder that you are blessed every day of your life.

Life is also different psychologically and emotionally. Your new normal might also include other changes, brought about by changes to your worldview. Think about all you've experienced: the depths of love and caring in others that you may not have witnessed before, your own wonder of waking up alive each morning, and the complete obliteration of ego and pride as you refocused your life lens on what truly matters. And while this can be a beautiful transformation of your own spirit, helping you develop clarity and renewed purpose, it might bring about the need for more patience with the world around you. Life continues to go on as it was before.

What am I talking about? When I was spending more time than usual resting, I'd pop the TV on and cringe seeing commercials for perfect hair, perfect skin, perfect teeth, and the perfect body, suddenly recognizing how superficial our culture has in many ways become. I mean, I had noticed before, but it was background noise that I just brushed off. But now that I could see things more clearly, I wanted to reach out to these companies and their audiences to explain that none of this matters. None of it. Our time is absolutely precious. What are we thinking?

So imagine my dismay when I went to a dinner party where an absolutely lovely 25-year-old woman matter-of-factly began describing the injections she gets into her forehead every six months to prevent wrinkles. I looked around the table hoping to see someone else as horrified as I was, but no. Just me. The conversation devolved further as she began evaluating every face at the table to determine the degree of "damage" the aging process had inflicted on each of us. She advised her dad that he should consider going with her to her next appointment for his own injections. He seemed to seriously contemplate the suggestion.

In the past, I would have watched this exchange with amusement. But the new me imploded. *What have we done to the next generation that they place such a high value on these valueless standards? Have we let them down completely?* I demanded of myself. *I hope it doesn't take a life-altering diagnosis to help these wonderful young souls recognize that they are perfect just the way they are and that they could be spending their efforts on much more meaningful pursuits.*

Patience, I reminded myself. Our new normal demands patience at every turn. Lucky for us, we developed a whole lot of that as we dealt with cancer. And maybe now that we have more clarity as well as patience, we can help change the world, as corny as that may sound, by sharing some of the lessons we've learned. I'm not saying that we're somehow smarter or better than anyone else, just that we might have some useful insights to share after all the time we've spent contemplating life and death, and what's truly important.

After doing this quick soul check-in, I tuned back in to the dinner conversation just in time to hear my date ask another guest, "So, Karen, what's the deal with Jennifer at your office? Wow, she's something. There's *no* way those can be real boobs — or *are* they?"

Well, fiddle-de-fucking-dee. Maybe we *are* smarter than some people! I won't get into the depth of sadness and disappointment this comment caused me, but I share it because you should prepare for people, sometimes even people you like or love, to occasionally say insensitive things. Of course they don't mean to be hurtful, but every now and then, a comment will hit a nerve like those zingers in your arm after surgery. *Ouch!* Lucky for you, you've developed that patient, calm spirit that will help you forgive and forget.

And when you do forgive and forget, just know that you're a better person than I am. Because I kicked that dude's can right to the curb. I couldn't help myself. I looked in the mirror and Tom's T-shirt looked back at me: *Who Has Time For This Shit?*

Chapter 16
Celebrate Life. Celebrate You!

Every day going forward is a gift.

When you get back to "normal" life, no matter how close or far that is from your previous "normal" life, never forget the important lessons you learned from cancer. Remember how you discovered your unbreakable spirit — your unshakable soul. Hold on to those moments when you looked into others and saw their beauty, maybe for the first time. Commit to making every new moment count. And celebrate yourself and your life every single day. Laugh! Hug someone! Hug yourself! Life is good, and you are awesome.

I've never been focused on keeping records of my achievements, but Rachel always remembers the exact date of my last treatment, and she reminds me every year that

WE DID IT! It's good to celebrate ourselves this way —
to acknowledge what we've been through and rejoice with
those who stood by our sides. It reminds us that every day
is a gift to be cherished.

When people ask me where cancer fits into my life
today, I explain that it's part of my fabric. Does it define
me? No. But I respect every minute of the journey and the
contributions it has made to who I am, what I hold dear,
and how I choose to go forward in life. I hope you will feel
this way, too, and recognize how much you have to give
the world — probably more than you ever imagined.

For example, think about the great potential you
hold to help those who are walking cancer's path behind
you. How gratifying would it be to reach back to lend
them a hand, sharing your own experiences and serving as
a role model? Having been through the rigors of cancer
yourself, you will feel so much more comfortable talking
with them, listening to their fears and feelings, and
assuring them that they have the strength within
themselves to weather any treatment, any pain, any
setback, any challenge. Show them how to celebrate the
victories, large and small, and remind them that they are

part of a caring, supportive community that has their back all the way.

As for you, remember that no matter what your prognosis may be, how your body may have changed, or what lasting symptoms you might experience, you should never *ever* give up on yourself. Ask for support when you need it, and don't let worry or fear hold you back from living the full life you deserve. In fact, live more freely, love more intensely, approach life more exuberantly, and drink in every moment.

We still have a lot of living to do, my friend. So today, let's dance in the street and not worry about who might be watching. Are we superheroes like the world may want to believe? Hell no. But we are bold, strong, beautiful flattops, ready to unleash our newfound badassery on the world. Who's with me? Grab that pink T-shirt and let's go!

www.ingramcontent.com/pod-product-compliance
Lightning Source LLC
LaVergne TN
LVHW021453080426
835509LV00018B/2264